# Keeping this book up to date

The page numbers given in the answers supplied herein relate to the page numbers in the first edition of the respective College Seminars book. As time goes by, each of these books will be superseded by a new edition. As that happens, a revised version of the relevant chapter of this book, drawn from and relating to the new edition, will be prepared and placed on the book's website at:

**www.rcpsych.ac.uk/publications/gaskell/89_7.htm**

We recommend that you check the website for the current updates before starting work on these questions.

In addition, certain titles in the series may go out of print and not merit reprinting because a new edition is imminent. The full text of such titles will also be made available on this site.

# College Seminars Series

## Series Editors

**Professor Hugh Freeman**, Honorary Professor, University of Salford, and Honorary Consultant Psychiatrist, Salford Health Authority

**Dr Ian Pullen**, Consultant Psychiatrist, Dingleton Hospital, Melrose, Roxburghshire

**Dr George Stein**, Consultant Psychiatrist, Farnborough Hospital, and King's College Hospital, London

**Professor Greg Wilkinson**, Editor, *British Journal of Psychiatry*, and Professor of Liaison Psychiatry, University of Liverpool

## About the author

**Dr David McNamara** is a specialist registrar in child and adolescent psychiatry at the Maudsley Hospital, London.

# Contents

# Preface

Writing the preface was the final task in the creation of this book, and was something that I had 'forgotten' in a Freudian sense. This book is not a pretension to a creative literary work but merely a distillation of the wisdom and knowledge of over 100 contributors to the College Seminars Series, whose work I have come to know intimately. This intimacy has only served to enhance the respect that I have for their work.

The extent of knowledge required to claim a grasp of both the art and science of psychiatry became apparent to me in the preparation of this book. I truly believe that MCQs are a valuable tool for consolidating the knowledge to be gleaned from the College Seminars Series, and I hope that these questions will be of benefit to those also striving to achieve an understanding of a complex, fascinating and profoundly rewarding medical speciality.

Many are justifiably anxious about MCQs. Faced with a bewildering range of potential topics, many will feel helpless. Some will argue that the process is random and warrants little attention. It is my contention that practising MCQs is, in fact, a superb preparation for knowledge consolidation. Not only does such practice direct one's learning to gaps in knowledge, but completing them helps to accrete knowledge.

The College Seminars Series provides a wide range of contemporary references to subspecialities of psychiatry and areas of basic science. These questions are filtered from those publications, many of which will be the only source of information at the requisite depth.

Whereas this book is single-authored, its genesis and production would not have been possible were it not for the tolerance of my wife, Melanie, and children, Holly, India and Elgin. I would also like to acknowledge the various editors of the series for providing current knowledge of each section and a particular gratitude to Dr George Stein for his mentoring role.

Every attempt has been made to minimise errors but inevitably flaws will surface. I welcome constructive criticism and suggestions.

# Alcohol and Drug Misuse

1　ICD–10 diagnostic criteria for psychoactive substance dependence include:

(a)　A minimum of four of the specified features.
(b)　Recurrent use in situations in which it is physically hazardous.
(c)　Tolerance.
(d)　Substance use to avoid withdrawal symptoms.
(e)　Narrowing of the personal repertoire of pattern of psychoactive substance use.

2　The following are true statements:

(a)　The reward effect of stimulants is mediated by the mesocortical and mesolimbic dopamine system.
(b)　Inhalation of volatile solvents is as common in girls as boys.
(c)　Codeine may give a morphine positive result on urine testing.
(d)　'Crack' is an unstable form of the freebase cocaine.
(e)　The most active constituent of cannabis is 9-tetrahydrocannabinol.

3　The following are Class A drugs:

(a)　Barbiturates.
(b)　Buprenorphine.
(c)　Phencyclidine.
(d)　Opium.
(e)　Intravenously administered amphetamines.

4　The following are psychological manifestations of sedative abstinence syndromes:

(a)　Profuse sweating.
(b)　Lethargy.
(c)　Insomnia.
(d)　Nightmares.
(e)　Dysphoria.

5　The following are physiological manifestations of sedative abstinence syndromes:

(a)　Shakiness.
(b)　Agitation.
(c)　Restlessness.
(d)　Impaired memory.
(e)　Concentration difficulties.

1   (a)  False (p. 2): three or more of seven experienced or exhibited at some
         time during the previous 12 months – a strong desire or sense of
         compulsion to take the substance; difficulties in controlling substance-
         taking behaviour in terms of its onset, termination or levels of use;
         a physiological withdrawal state when substance use has ceased or
         been reduced; evidence of tolerance; progressive neglect of alternative
         pleasures or interests because of psychoactive substance use;
         persisting with substance use despite clear evidence of overtly harmful
         consequences; narrowing of the personal repertoire of patterns of
         psychoactive substance use has also been described as a characteristic
         feature.
     (b)  False (p. 2): this is a DSM–IV criterion.
     (c)  True (p. 3).
     (d)  True (p. 3).
     (e)  True (p. 3).

2   (a)  True (p. 21).
     (b)  True (p. 27).
     (c)  True (p. 37).
     (d)  False (p. 47): it is a stable form of the freebase cocaine.
     (e)  True (p. 49).

3   (a)  False (p. 36): Class B.
     (b)  False (p. 36): Class C.
     (c)  True (p. 36).
     (d)  True (p. 36).
     (e)  True (p. 36): Class A drugs – cocaine, LSD, phencyclidine,
         diamorphine, morphine, methadone, pethidine, opium, dextro-
         moramide, dipipanone, alfentanil, and class B drugs when prepared
         for injection. Class B includes oral amphetamines, barbiturates,
         cannabis and some opiates. Class C includes most benzodiazepines,
         buprenorphine and a variety of other drugs deemed liable to misuse.

4   (a)  False (p. 57): physiological.
     (b)  False (p. 57): physiological.
     (c)  True (p. 57).
     (d)  True (p. 57).
     (e)  True (p. 57).

5   (a)  True (p. 57).
     (b)  False (p. 57): psychological.
     (c)  False (p. 57): psychological.
     (d)  False (p. 57): psychological.
     (e)  False (p. 57): psychological.

6   In the differential diagnosis of physical dependence and recurrent anxiety in relation to withdrawal of medium- to long-acting benzodiazepines, the following are true:
(a)   Physical dependency symptoms present earlier.
(b)   Recurrent anxiety symptoms reach maximum intensity at one week.
(c)   Recurrent anxiety symptoms typically present with new symptoms.
(d)   Physical dependency symptoms often include flu-like symptoms.
(e)   Physical dependency symptoms reduce after 14 days.


7   The following are correct statements with reference to benzodiazepines:
(a)   The higher the dose, the more likely it is that the patient will experience withdrawal symptoms.
(b)   There is a shorter time frame for the development of withdrawal symptoms when higher doses are administered.
(c)   The time of onset after withdrawal is less after a sudden withdrawal of short-acting benzodiazepines.
(d)   The risk of abstinence symptoms is greater in patients with chronic dysphoric states.
(e)   Those with obsessional personality are less likely to show symptoms on withdrawal.


8   Caffeinism:
(a)   Withdrawal syndrome starts after 48 hours.
(b)   Withdrawal syndrome lasts up to 1 week.
(c)   Caffeine has a half-life of 12 hours.
(d)   Caffeinism can precipitate panic attacks.
(e)   Muscle relaxation is a feature.


9   The following are true statements of the biological markers of vulnerability to alcoholism:
(a)   Enhanced response to thyrotropin-releasing hormone (TRH).
(b)   Increased alpha activity on electroencephalography (EEG).
(c)   Increased static ataxia.
(d)   Hyper-reactive autonomic nervous system.
(e)   Reduced amplitude and latency of the P300 event-related potential (ERP).


10   With reference to the aetiology of alcoholism:
(a)   50% of Chinese people possess a deficiency of aldehyde decarboxylase.
(b)   Aldehyde dehydrogenase (ALDH) activity is increased in alcoholics.
(c)   In operant conditioning neutral stimuli may become associated with drinking and become conditioned stimuli leading to craving.
(d)   Hyperactivity in childhood has been associated.
(e)   Alcoholism has been found to be associated with borderline personality disorder.

6   (a)  True  (p. 59): onset is in 2–3 days; with recurrent anxiety onset is in
         7 days.
     (b)  False (p. 59): physical dependency maximum is reached in 7–8 days
         (reduces in 14 days) and recurrent anxiety reaches a maximum in
         14+ days and continues.
     (c)  False (p. 59): old symptoms.
     (d)  True  (p. 59).
     (e)  True  (p. 59).

7   (a)  True  (p. 60).
     (b)  True  (p. 60).
     (c)  True  (p. 60).
     (d)  True  (p. 60).
     (e)  True  (p. 60): suggestion by Marks and by Woods *et al.*

8   (a)  False (p. 72): 12–24 hours.
     (b)  True  (p. 72).
     (c)  False (p. 72): 3–6 hours.
     (d)  True  (p. 73).
     (e)  False (p. 73): muscle tension.

9   (a)  True  (p. 97).
     (b)  False (p. 97): reduced.
     (c)  True  (p. 97).
     (d)  True  (p. 97).
     (e)  False (p. 97): increased latency, reduced amplitude.

10  (a)  False (p. 104): aldehyde dehydrogenase.
     (b)  False (p. 106): reduced activity of aldehyde dehydrogenase.
     (c)  False (p. 107): this is classical conditioning.
     (d)  True  (p. 109).
     (e)  True  (p. 111).

11  The following are true statements:
(a)  The CAGE questionnaire is a four-question screening item.
(b)  Elevated gamma-glutamyltransferase (GGT) normalises within 1–3 weeks with abstinence.
(c)  Mean cell volume (MCV) normalises quicker than GGT.
(d)  Carbohydrate-deficient transferrin (CDT) is less accurate as a marker of alcohol problems in women than men.
(e)  CDT has a lower false positive rate than either GGT or MCV.

12  The following features are guidelines for agreeing a goal of controlled drinking as opposed to abstinence:
(a)  Age greater than 40 years.
(b)  Impulsive traits.
(c)  Poor social support.
(d)  Evident dependence.
(e)  Abnormal liver functioning.

13  Disulfiram:
(a)  Disulfiram ('Antabuse') may be regarded as a form of exposure/response prevention therapy.
(b)  Disulfiram acts by inhibiting alcohol dehydrogenase.
(c)  Inhibition caused by disulfiram is irreversible.
(d)  Disulfiram should not be commenced within 3 days of alcohol consumption.
(e)  Alcohol should be avoided for 3 days following cessation of disulfiram.

14  Relative contraindications to disulfiram include:
(a)  Thyroid disease.
(b)  Epilepsy.
(c)  Antihypertensive medication.
(d)  Diabetes mellitus.
(e)  Psychosis.

15  With reference to the steps in the process of behaviour change as per Prochaska & DiClemente:
(a)  In 'pre-contemplation' individuals are considering change.
(b)  In 'preparation for change' individuals may still be ambivalent about their behaviour.
(c)  The 'contemplation' stage is characterised by awareness of costs and benefits of behaviour.
(d)  'Action' is the stage at which individuals make a firm resolution to change.
(e)  'Relapse prevention' is the final stage described.

11   (a)  True  (p. 130).
     (b)  True  (p. 130).
     (c)  False (p. 130): 2–10 weeks.
     (d)  True  (p. 130): CDT is positive in 80% of men admitting to problems
          with alcohol.
     (e)  True  (p. 130): that is, it has high sensitivity and specificity.

12   (a)  False (p. 137): age greater than 40 is a guideline for agreeing a goal
          of abstinence.
     (b)  False (p. 137): No impulsive traits is a guideline for agreeing goals
          of controlled drinking.
     (c)  False (p. 137): poor social support is a guideline for agreeing a goal
          of abstinence.
     (d)  False (p. 137): similarly, abstinence.
     (e)  False (p. 137): similarly, abstinence.

13   (a)  True  (p. 144).
     (b)  False (p. 144): aldehyde dehydrogenase.
     (c)  True  (p. 144).
     (d)  False (p. 145): 24 hours.
     (e)  False (p. 145): 1 week.

14   (a)  False (p. 146): this is a contraindication to calcium carbimide.
     (b)  True  (p. 146).
     (c)  True  (p. 146).
     (d)  True  (p. 146).
     (e)  True  (p. 146).

15   (a)  False (p. 159): relatively content with their behaviour.
     (b)  False (p. 159): involved in planning of behaviour change.
     (c)  True  (p. 159).
     (d)  False (p. 159): they make an initial attempt to modify problematic
          behaviour.
     (e)  False (p. 159): maintenance is the final stage described.

16   Features of delirium tremens include:
(a)   Autonomic overarousal.
(b)   Delusions.
(c)   Mood instability.
(d)   Hypnogogic hallucinations.
(e)   Pyrexia.

17   With regard to psychosis induced by illicit substances the following are true:
(a)   Stereotypical movements are a common feature of amphetamine psychosis.
(b)   Khat induces a temporary amphetamine-like psychosis.
(c)   Violence is sometimes a feature of heavy cocaine intake.
(d)   The prognosis of hallucinogenic psychosis is satisfactory.
(e)   Cannabis exacerbates pre-existing schizophrenia.

18   Alcoholic hallucinosis is characterised by:
(a)   Preservation or only slight clouding of consciousness.
(b)   Second person auditory hallucinations.
(c)   Bizarre delusions.
(d)   Clear link with alcohol withdrawal.
(e)   Thought disorder.

19   Cerebral damage in alcoholism:
(a)   Brain shrinkage is attributable to brain white matter changes.
(b)   White matter changes can be reversible.
(c)   Sulcal widening is commonly seen on computed tomography brains in attenders at alcohol problem clinics.
(d)   Radiological changes are partial reversible in the course of months of abstinence.
(e)   General intelligence is little affected on psychometric testing.

20   Areas of the brain implicated in Wernicke–Korsakoff syndrome include:
(a)   Paraventricular parts of the thalamus.
(b)   Paraventricular parts of the hypothalamus.
(c)   Periaquaductal grey matter of the midbrain.
(d)   Walls of fourth ventricle.
(e)   Superior colliculi.

21   In Korsakoff's psychosis the following are features:
(a)   Consciousness and perception are unaltered.
(b)   Disturbances of affect.
(c)   Disturbances of volition.
(d)   Patients are distressed by their memory impairment.
(e)   Abulia.

16  (a)  True (p. 175).
    (b)  True (p. 175).
    (c)  True (p. 175).
    (d)  True (p. 174): they include hypnogogic and hypnopompic hallucinations.
    (e)  True (p. 175).

17  (a)  True (p. 177): following prolonged consumption of large amounts of the drug.
    (b)  True (p. 178).
    (c)  True (p. 178).
    (d)  True (p. 179).
    (e)  True (p. 179).

18  (a)  True (p. 180).
    (b)  False (p. 180): usually refer to patient in third person.
    (c)  False (p. 180): not bizarre – often take the form of secondary delusions that attempt to explain hallucinations.
    (d)  False (p. 180): no clear link with alcohol withdrawal.
    (e)  False (p. 180).

19  (a)  True (p. 182).
    (b)  True (p. 182): unlike lesions of cortical neurons.
    (c)  True (p. 182).
    (d)  True (p. 183).
    (e)  True (p. 183).

20  (a)  True (p. 185).
    (b)  True (p. 185).
    (c)  True (p. 185).
    (d)  False (p. 185): it includes the floor but not the walls of the fourth ventricle.
    (e)  False (p. 185): it includes mammillary bodies.

21  (a)  True (p. 186).
    (b)  True (p. 186).
    (c)  True (p. 186).
    (d)  False (p. 186).
    (e)  True (p. 186): patients are content to spend their time virtually unoccupied; there is also preservation of verbal performance and social skills.

22  The following are true statements regarding alcoholic liver disease:
(a)  Peak incidence of alcoholic liver cirrhosis is at 30–45 years.
(b)  70% of patients attending alcohol treatment units in the UK have abnormal liver histology.
(c)  Fatty liver can lead to liver failure and jaundice.
(d)  The most reliable indicators of poor hepatic function are the serum transaminases.
(e)  The 5-year survival following diagnosis of alcoholic cirrhosis is good.

23  The following are associated with regular heavy drinking:
(a)  Peripheral neuropathy occurs in 20% of heavy drinkers.
(b)  Worsening of psoriasis.
(c)  Avascular necrosis of the femoral head.
(d)  Alcoholic cardiomyopathy, usually presenting as arrhythmia.
(e)  Resistance to osteoporosis in men.

24  Foetal alcohol syndrome is based on the presence of:
(a)  Prenatal growth retardation.
(b)  Developmental delay.
(c)  Macrocephaly.
(d)  Prominent upper lip.
(e)  Prominent maxillary area.

22   (a)  False (p. 202): 40–55 years.
     (b)  True  (p. 202).
     (c)  False (p. 203): it is benign and reversible.
     (d)  False (p. 204): raised prothrombin time and low serum albumin.
     (e)  True  (p. 204): the majority of patients who abstain are alive.

23   (a)  False (p. 207): 10% of very heavy drinkers.
     (b)  True  (p. 208).
     (c)  True  (p. 208).
     (d)  False (p. 209): cardiac failure.
     (e)  False (p.208): in post-menopausal women, moderate alcohol
          consumption may delay development of osteoperosis.

24   (a)  True  (p. 217): also postnatal growth retardation.
     (b)  True  (p. 217): also intellectual impairment.
     (c)  False (p. 217): microcephaly.
     (d)  False (p. 217): thin upper lip.
     (e)  False (p. 217): flat maxillary area.

# Clinical Psychopharmacology

1  The following are true in relation to transmitters:
(a) Dale's law states that for each neuron the same transmitter is released at all its synapses.
(b) A neurotransmitter must be present in a nerve terminal and in the vicinity of the area of the brain where it is thought to act to fulfil definition criteria.
(c) A neurotransmitter should be released from the nerve terminal following nerve stimulation.
(d) A neurotransmitter should activate a postsynaptic receptor site following its release.
(e) The enzymes concerned in the synthesis and metabolism of meurotransmitters should be present in the nerve ending.

2  The 'depolarisation' process involves the following:
(a) Depolarisation opens potassium channels.
(b) The falling phase of the action potential is caused by closing of sodium channels.
(c) In all nerve cells action potentials are followed by a transient hyper-polarisation.
(d) During the refractory period it is impossible to trigger an action potential.
(e) All excitatory neurotransmitters produce excitatory postsynaptic potentials.

3  The following are correct:
(a) The major inhibitory transmitters are gamma-aminobutyric acid (GABA) and glycine.
(b) Dopamine is inhibitory on $D_1$ and $D_5$ receptors.
(c) Acetylcholine has excitatory and inhibitory properties.
(d) Adrenaline's distribution in the brain is mainly in the midbrain and brain-stem.
(e) Glutamate is implicated in learning and memory.

4  The following are correct statements:
(a) Tetrodotoxin selectively blocks potassium channels.
(b) Drugs which selectively block potassium channels may have therapeutic uses in multiple sclerosis.
(c) The $D_2$ dopamine receptor inhibits the activity of adenylate cyclase.
(d) Presynaptic inhibition is restricted to noradrenergic and GABA-ergic synapses.
(e) Some adrenoceptor antagonists such as phentolamine enhance the release of the noradrenaline.

11

1   (a) True (p. 1): Dale's law applies only to the presynaptic portion of the neuron, not the postsynaptic effects which the transmitter may have on other target neurons.
    (b) True (p. 2).
    (c) True (p. 2): generally by a calcium-dependent process; again, this statement refers to criteria which must be fulfilled for a substance to be considered as a transmitter.
    (d) True (p. 2).
    (e) True (p. 2): or in the proximity of the nerve ending.

    Note. These criteria should be regarded as general guidelines, not specific rules.

2   (a) False (p. 4): sodium channels open, allowing an increase in sodium ion influx into the cell, producing the rising phase of the action potential.
    (b) True (p. 4): which reduces the influx of sodium ions.
    (c) False (p. 4): in most nerve cells but not all.
    (d) False (p. 4): only possible if the stimulus is stronger than normal.
    (e) True (p. 4): which last for approximately 5 ms.

3   (a) True (p. 5).
    (b) False (p. 3): Inhibitory on $D_2$ and stimulatory on $D_1$ and $D_5$
    (c) True (p. 3): excitatory on $M_1$ and N receptors and inhibitory on $M_2$ receptors.
    (d) True (p. 3).
    (e) False (p. 3): glycine.

4   (a) False (p. 5): it selectively blocks sodium channels and thus paralyses conduction.
    (b) True (p. 5).
    (c) True (p. 6): $D_1$ receptors stimulate adenylate cyclase and $D_2$ receptors inhibit adenylate cyclase.
    (d) False (p. 8): presynaptic inhibition occurs in noradrenergic and GABA-ergic synapses and also in dopaminergic and serotonergic synapses.
    (e) False (p. 8): some adrenoceptor antagonists such as phenoxybenzamine enhance the release of the amine.

5    Dopamine receptors:

(a)   The $D_2$ receptor is negatively linked with adenylate cyclase.
(b)   The $D_1$ receptor is approximately 15 times more sensitive to the action of dopamine than the $D_2$ receptor.
(c)   $D_2$ receptors are located presynaptically on the corticostriatal neurons and postsynaptically in the striatum and substantia nigra.
(d)   $D_4$ receptor density is highest in basal ganglia.
(e)   Clozapine has a selective affinity for $D_5$ receptors.


6    With reference to serotonin (5-hydroxytryptamine; 5-HT) receptors the following are true:

(a)   The selective agonist of $5\text{-HT}_{1A}$ receptor is 8-hydroxydipropylamino-tetralin (8-OH-DPAT).
(b)   $5\text{-HT}_2$ receptors appear to mediate excitatory effects particularly in the cortex.
(c)   Ritanserin is a specific antagonist for $5\text{-HT}_2$ receptors.
(d)   Ondansetron is a $5\text{-HT}_3$ receptor antagonist.
(e)   $5\text{-HT}_2$ receptors are found in concentrations in the claustrum.


7    With regard to amino acid receptors the following are true:

(a)   Benzodiazepines occupy a receptor site on the GABA receptor complex.
(b)   Glycine acts on the N-methyl-D-aspartate (NMDA) receptor.
(c)   The $GABA_A$ receptor is directly linked with chloride ion channels.
(d)   Cyclopyrrolone sedatives increase the frequency of chloride ion channel opening.
(e)   Flumazenil blocks the action of agonist on the $GABA_B$ receptor.


8    The following are true with reference to excitatory amino acid receptors:

(a)   NMDA receptor activity is modulated by chloride ions.
(b)   Phencyclidine ('angel dust') acts as an agonist at the NMDA-linked ion channel.
(c)   NMDA receptors are found in high concentrations in the Raphe nuclei.
(d)   Epilepsy may occur as a result of sudden release of glycine.
(e)   Neuronal death due to the toxic effects of glutamate has been implicated in cerebral ischaemia.


9    In pharmacokinetics the following are true statements:

(a)   First-order kinetics means a non-reversible reaction proceeds at an ever increasing rate as the amount of the reacting substance falls.
(b)   Alcohol follows zero-order kinetics.
(c)   The concentration of an intravenously administered drug declines in an exponential fashion.
(d)   Bioavailability refers to the fraction of drug that has been metabolised.
(e)   Two dosage forms of the same drug with an equal bioavailability are not necessarily bioequivalent.

5   (a)  True (p. 15): $D_1$ is positively linked.
    (b)  True (p. 15).
    (c)  True (p. 15): $D_1$ receptors are found presynaptically on nigrostriatal neurons and postsynaptically in the cortex.
    (d)  False (p. 16): frontal cortex and amygdala.
    (e)  False (p. 17): $D_4$.

6   (a)  True (p. 18).
    (b)  True (p. 18).
    (c)  True (p. 18): ritanserin is a specific antagonist for $5\text{-}HT_2$ receptors and has anxiolytic properties.
    (d)  True (p. 18).
    (e)  True (p. 19): $5\text{-}HT_2$ receptors are concentrated in the claustrum and cortex and olfactory system.

7   (a)  True (p. 20): which enhances the responsiveness of the GABA receptor to the inhibitory effects of GABA.
    (b)  True (p. 20).
    (c)  True (p. 20).
    (d)  True (p. 21): e.g. zopiclone.
    (e)  False (p. 21): $GABA_A$.

8   (a)  False (p. 23): NMDA receptors are widely distributed in the brain and their activity is modulated by magnesium ions.
    (b)  False (p. 23): phencyclidine and ketamine block the NMDA-linked ion channel.
    (c)  False (p. 24): the hippocampus and cortex.
    (d)  False (p. 24): glutamate.
    (e)  True (p. 24): associated with multi-infarct dementia.

9   (a)  False (p. 28): the majority of drugs follow first-order kinetics, where the rate of absorption depends on the dose remaining to be absorbed and the rate of elimination directly depends on the amount of drug remaining in the body. Zero-order kinetics describes processes where the rate of absorption is independent of the concentration of the drug, e.g. the absorption of a drug from a slow-release preparation, the slow infusion of a drug or the elimination of some drugs such as alcohol and phenytoin because of rapid saturation of metabolising enzymes.
    (b)  True (pp. 28–29).
    (c)  True (p. 29): follows first-order kinetics.
    (d)  False (p. 30): bioavailability refers to the fraction of drug 'that has been absorbed'. Bioequivalence is dependent upon efficacy, which in turn depends on plasma concentration.
    (e)  True (p. 30).

10   With reference to pharmacokinetics the following are true:

(a)   Drugs with large distribution volumes will invariably reach the transcellular regions such as the brain and foetus.
(b)   Phenylbutazone has a similar volume of distribution to the plasma volume.
(c)   Haloperidol possesses a volume of distribution of greater than 2 l/kg.
(d)   Dopamine, unlike levo-dopa, is able to cross the blood–brain barrier.
(e)   The therapeutic window is the range of plasma concentrations which yields therapeutic success.

11   The following are true of the pharmacokinetics of benzodiazepines:

(a)   When long acting they have a long elimination half-life.
(b)   When short acting they have a small distribution volume.
(c)   When long acting they have no active metabolites.
(d)   When short acting they have minimal accumulation.
(e)   Benzodiazepines with a half-life of 12 hours tend to be used as anxiolytics.

12   The effects of drugs on human performance can be measured by a range of tests. The following are true statements with reference to this statement.

(a)   Assessment of sensory function is by the critical flicker fusion (CFF) threshold.
(b)   Paper and pencil tests, such as digit symbol substitution, measure central nervous system (CNS) arousal.
(c)   Stabilometer devices measure sensory function.
(d)   The Gibson spiral maze test measures CNS arousal.
(e)   The card-sorting test measures motor function.

13   The following conditions usually show a marked non-drug-specific (placebo) response and/or sustained spontaneous recovery:

(a)   Adjustment disorders.
(b)   Dissociative states.
(c)   Drug-induced psychosis.
(d)   Major depressive episodes.
(e)   Manic episodes.

10 (a) True (p. 32).
   (b) True (p. 32): reflects the drug's strong affinity for plasma proteins.
   (c) True (p. 32).
   (d) False (p. 34): the reverse is true: levo-dopa crosses the blood–brain barrier, unlike dopamine. The blood–brain barrier behaves as an extreme form of lipid membrane highly selective for lipid-soluble molecules. Lipophilic drugs pass in both directions between plasma water and the brain, usually by passive diffusion.
   (e) True (p. 39): the size of this depends on the ratio of maximum tolerated concentration (MTC) and minimum effective concentration (MEC), or therapeutic index.

11 (a) True (p. 42).
   (b) False (p. 42): they have a high distribution volume.
   (c) False (p. 42): when short acting they have no active metabolites.
   (d) True (p. 42).
   (e) False (p. 42): hypnotics have a short half-life (8–12 hours) – anxiolytics tend to have a half-life in the region of 40–100 hours.

   Note. Long-acting benzodiazepines have a long elimination half-life, small distribution volume, accumulation, active metabolites and residual effects. Short-acting benzodiazepines have a short elimination half-life, higher distribution volume, minimal accumulation and no active metabolites.

12 (a) False (p. 54): changes in CNS arousal are often measured by means of the CFF, which exploits the phenomenon that a decrease in arousal of the CNS is accompanied by a fall in the maximum flickering frequency of a light that can be detected.
   (b) False (p. 54): this assesses sensory function, recognition or perception.
   (c) False (p. 54): these assess motor function and balance. Other measures of ballistic activity include finger tapping.
   (d) False (p. 54): this assesses sensorimotor function. Other examples which assess sensorimotor function include the pursuit rotor test, card sorting, reaction time and the measurement of saccadic eye movements.
   (e) False (p. 54): this assesses sensorimotor function.

13 (a) True (p. 67).
   (b) True (p. 67).
   (c) True (p. 67).
   (d) True (p. 67): placebo responses may occur early in treatment but are often not sustained.
   (e) True (p. 67).

   Note. Additionally, anxiety disorders, conversion states, reactive mood disorders.

14 The following show low placebo response:
(a) Dysthymia.
(b) Residual symptoms of chronic schizophrenia.
(c) Obsessive–compulsive disorder.
(d) Chronic anxiety disorder.
(e) Conversion states.

15 All trials in a meta-analysis should satisfy minimum standards for:
(a) Random allocation of patients.
(b) Blind assessment.
(c) Measurements.
(d) Outcome criteria.
(e) Treatment variables.

16 Depressive symptoms indicating a favourable response to anti-depressant drugs include:
(a) Reduced appetite.
(b) Late insomnia.
(c) Evening worsening of mood.
(d) Anhedonia.
(e) Motor agitation.

17 The nocebo effect entails:
(a) Overcoming negative attitudes to drug treatment.
(b) Increasing expectations of drug treatment.
(c) Patients thinking they are being deprived of something which they believe will benefit them.
(d) Amplification of adverse responses to treatment withdrawal.
(e) Making the patient feel as much at ease as possible.

18 The following are correctly paired:
(a) Anorgasmia as a side-effect of selective serotonin reuptake inhibitors (SSRIs) may be treated with a 5-HT blocker.
(b) Excess sweating associated with tricyclic antidepressants may be treated with an alpha$_1$ blocker.
(c) Polyuria associated with lithium may be treated with carbamazepine.
(d) Leucopenia associated with carbamazepine may be treated with lithium.
(e) Impaired ejaculation associated with tricyclic antidepressants may be treated with neostigmine.

14  (a)  True (p. 68).
    (b)  True (p. 68).
    (c)  True (p. 68).
    (d)  True (p. 68).
    (e)  False (p. 67): usually shows marked placebo response.

15  (a)  True (p. 76).
    (b)  True (p. 76).
    (c)  True (p. 76).
    (d)  True (p. 76).
    (e)  True (p. 76): trials cannot be identical and are likely to have used slightly different patient groups or treatment variables.

    Note. Meta-analysis comprises a group of techniques for objectively and systematically pooling the results of controlled trials which have investigated similar hypotheses concerning the efficacy of particular treatments. All trials should be included, not just those giving positive results.

16  (a)  True (p. 81).
    (b)  True (p. 81): also mid insomnia.
    (c)  False (p. 81): morning worsening of mood.
    (d)  True (p. 81).
    (e)  True (p. 81).

    Note. Aditionally, weight loss, distinct quality of altered mood, motor retardation, hopelessness and guilt.

17  (a)  False (pp. 87–88): the doctor overcoming negative attitudes to drug treatment helps to produce a placebo effect. Conversely, increasing negative attitudes and expectations represent a nocebo component of treatment.
    (b)  True (p. 88).
    (c)  True (p. 88).
    (d)  True (p. 88).
    (e)  True (p. 87): this helps to produce a placebo effect.

18  (a)  True (p. 91): anorgasmia as a side-effect of SSRIs may be treated with a 5-HT blocker such as cyproheptidine.
    (b)  True (p. 91): excess sweating associated with tricyclic antidepressants may be treated with an $alpha_1$ blocker such as terazocin.
    (c)  True (p. 91): polyuria associated with lithium may be treated with carbamazepine, which is an antidiuretic hormone sensitiser.
    (d)  True (p. 91).
    (e)  True (p. 91): impaired ejaculation and reduced libido may be treated with anticholinesterases such as neostigmine.

19 The principal neurotransmitter systems implicated in anxiety are:

(a) Acetylcholine.
(b) Noradrenaline.
(c) Glycine.
(d) GABA.
(e) Serotonin.

20 Barbiturates have the following characteristics:

(a) Thiobarbiturates are highly protein bound and highly lipid soluble.
(b) Orally administered barbiturates are less protein bound than those given intravenously.
(c) Barbiturates inhibit hepatic microsomal enzymes.
(d) Elimination half-lives are in the range of 30–90 hours for long-acting barbiturates.
(e) Orally administered barbiturates are metabolised quickly but have a longer duration of action.

21 Barbiturates have the following features:

(a) They enhance the action of GABA at its receptors.
(b) The main adverse effects are on psychomotor function.
(c) They inhibit their own metabolism.
(d) Tolerance and dependence both develop rapidly.
(e) In children attention deficit hyperactivity disorder (ADHD) may occur with their use.

22 The GABA receptor complex has the following features:

(a) $GABA_B$ receptors are involved in mediating the effects of barbiturates.
(b) The effects of GABA are sometimes excitatory.
(c) Chloride channels open when GABA binds to a postsynaptic $GABA_A$ receptor.
(d) Benzodiazepine receptors are separate from GABA receptors.
(e) GABA binds to benzodiazepine receptors.

23 The following are true of receptor ligands:

(a) An agonist has the characteristic effect at the receptor of the 'normal' transmitter substance.
(b) In the case of benzodiazepine receptors 'inverse' agonists are anticonvulsants.
(c) Full agonists at the benzodiazepine receptor appear to enhance the binding of GABA to its receptors.
(d) Competitive antagonists block the effects of both agonists and antagonists.
(e) Flumazenil is an antagonist and also has potential inverse agonist effects.

19  (a)  False (p. 103).
    (b)  True (p. 103).
    (c)  False (p. 103).
    (d)  True (p. 103).
    (e)  True (p. 103).

20  (a)  True (p. 104): e.g. thiopental intravenously.
    (b)  True (p. 104): also less lipid soluble.
    (c)  False (p. 104): they are hepatic enzyme inducers.
    (d)  True (p. 104).
    (e)  False (p. 104): they are metabolised slowly, they are also less protein bound and less lipid soluble.

21  (a)  True (p. 105).
    (b)  True (p. 105): cognitive performance and motor skills are both impaired. Other adverse effects are vertigo, nausea, vomiting and diarrhoea.
    (c)  False (p. 105): they are inducers.
    (d)  True (p. 105).
    (e)  False (p. 105): but paradoxical hyperactivity may occur.

22  (a)  False (p. 106): $GABA_A$ mediates the effects of benzodiazepines and barbiturates.
    (b)  False (p. 106): inhibitory.
    (c)  True (p. 106).
    (d)  True (p. 108).
    (e)  False (p. 108): GABA and benzodiazepine receptors are separate.

23  (a)  True (p. 109).
    (b)  False (p. 110): they are convulsant and anxiogenic. Inverse agonists have the opposite effect to agonists.
    (c)  True (p. 110).
    (d)  False (p. 110): they block the effects of agonists and inverse agonists.
    (e)  True (p. 110): antagonist to diazepam and slight partial inverse agonist effects leading to anxiogenic features, primarily in patients with panic disorder.

24   Diazepam has the following pharmacokinetic properties:

(a)   An elimination half-life which is 10 times greater in elderly than young adults.
(b)   50% bioavailability with an oral dose.
(c)   50% protein binding.
(d)   An inactive metabolite, desmethyldiazepam.
(e)   The presence of food reduces the extent of absorption.


25   Occasional adverse effects of diazepam include:

(a)   Amnesia.
(b)   Restlessness.
(c)   Skin rash.
(d)   Psychomotor impairment.
(e)   Dizziness.


26   The following physiological effects are noted for benzodiazepines:

(a)   At normal therapeutic doses benzodiazepines have little effect on autonomic function.
(b)   Benzodiazepines induce hepatic microsomal enzymes.
(c)   The dexamethasone suppression test is usually unaffected.
(d)   Inhibition of afferent pathways in the spinal cord results in skeletal muscle relaxation.
(e)   Neuroendocrine measures are not affected.


27   The following comparisons of benzodiazepine properties are true:

(a)   Lorazepam has a higher receptor affinity than oxazepam.
(b)   Diazepam is a more highly lipid-soluble drug than lorazepam.
(c)   Lorazepam is highly water soluble.
(d)   Alprazolam's half-life determines doses be given at least three times daily.
(e)   Flurazepam has a long half-life and accumulates.


28   Hepatic enzyme inducers include:

(a)   Phenytoin.
(b)   Carbamazepine.
(c)   Isoniazid.
(d)   Rifampicin.
(e)   Cimetidine.


29   Flumazenil has the following properties:

(a)   It is a partial antagonist at benzodiazepine receptors.
(b)   Agitation is a side-effect.
(c)   Occasionally it is epileptogenic.
(d)   It has a long elimination half-life.
(e)   It is useful in panic disorder.

24   (a)   False (p. 113): in young adults it is approximately 20 hours and in
the elderly it is between 30 and 100 hours.
(b)   False (p. 113): almost complete bioavailability with an oral dose.
(c)   False (p. 113): 95% protein bound.
(d)   False (p. 114): it is an active metabolite.
(e)   False (p. 113): it reduces the rate but not the extent.

25   (a)   False (p. 114): rare.
(b)   False (p. 114): rare.
(c)   False (p. 114): rare.
(d)   False (p. 114): common.
(e)   False (p. 114): common.

> Note. Occasional adverse effects include dry mouth, blurred vision,
> gastrointestinal upset, ataxia, headache and hypotension.

26   (a)   True (p. 115): also, at normal therapeutic doses, they have little effect
on cardiovascular or respiratory function, although they may sometimes cause respiratory depression and reduce systolic blood pressure.
(b)   False (p. 115).
(c)   True (p. 115): but chronic high-dose therapy may interfere with
dexamethasone supression.
(d)   True (p. 115).
(e)   True (p. 115): usually unchanged, although occasionally plasma
cortisol may be decreased.

27   (a)   True (p. 116): lorazepam also has a higher affinity than diazepam.
(b)   True (p. 117): rapidly absorbed and rapidly reaches the brain.
(c)   True (p. 118).
(d)   True (p. 118).
(e)   False (p. 118): the parent drug has a short half-life (2 hours) but
active metabolites have a long half-life, of 36–120 hours.

28   (a)   True (p. 119).
(b)   True (p. 119).
(c)   False (p. 119): inhibits.
(d)   True (p. 119).
(e)   False (p. 119): inhibits.

29   (a)   False (p. 120): it is an antagonist and partial inverse agonist at
benzodiazepine receptors.
(b)   True (p. 120): also anxiety and nausea.
(c)   True (p. 120).
(d)   False (p. 120): a short elimination half-life, of 1–2 hours.
(e)   False (p. 110): it aggravates panic disorder.

> Note. The short elimination half-life has the clinical implication that it is necessary
> to continue monitoring until the plasma benzodiazepine levels fall to below
> dangerous levels.

30 Neurophysiology of sleep:
(a) Wakefulness is maintained by activity of the ascending reticular activating system.
(b) The onset of sleep is due to a decrease in reticular activating system activity.
(c) Approximately 25% of total sleep time is made up of rapid eye movement.
(d) High frequency, 12–14 Hz, sleep spindles occur in stage II.
(e) In the elderly stage IV and total sleep time decreases.

31 Effects of hypnotics on sleep:
(a) Benzodiazepines suppress stage IV sleep.
(b) With chronic benzodiazepine use suppression of REM sleep in the early part of the night occurs.
(c) On withdrawal of benzodiazepines a rebound increase above the 'normal' amount of REM sleep occurs.
(d) It may take up to 6 weeks to see a return to a normal sleep pattern on benzodiazepine withdrawal.
(e) Barbiturates are more likely to suppress REM sleep than are benzodiazepines.

32 Tolerance to benzodiazepine effects occurs in the following situations:
(a) Tolerance develops to the ataxic but not muscle-relaxant properties.
(b) Tolerance to the anticonvulsant properties develops slowly.
(c) Tolerance develops to auditory evoked responses.
(d) Tachyphylaxis may develop to the sedative effects.
(e) Tolerance is more likely to develop to anxiolysis than sedation.

33 Rare features of the benzodiazepine withdrawal syndrome include:
(a) Hallucinations.
(b) Seizures.
(c) Paranoid psychosis.
(d) Confusional states.
(e) Hyperacusis.

30   (a)   True (p. 120).
     (b)   False (p. 120): it is due to activity arising from other midbrain centres, particularly the Raphe nuclei and locus coeruleus.
     (c)   True (p. 121).
     (d)   True (p. 120).
     (e)   True (p. 121).

Note. Table 4.4. on p. 121 provides a useful summary of sleep stages.

31   (a)   True (p. 122): also suppress REM sleep.
     (b)   False (p. 122): in the early stage REM suppression occurs but tolerance develops with chronic use.
     (c)   True (p. 122): on withdrawal of the drug the normal physiological drive to induce REM sleep is unmasked (having been inhibited by the drug) and adds to the increased drive that has developed during the process of tolerance – this resuts in more dreaming, nightmares and nocturnal awakenings.
     (d)   True (p. 122).
     (e)   True (p. 122).

32   (a)   False (p. 123): develops to both ataxic and muscle-relaxant properties, as well as anticonvulsant properties.
     (b)   False (p. 123): tolerance develops rapidly, so benzodiazepines are of little value in long-term prophylaxis.
     (c)   True (p. 123).
     (d)   True (p. 124): that is, very rapid tolerance.
     (e)   False (p. 125): tolerance to sedation is greater than that to psycho-motor or amnestic effects, which is also greater than that to anxiolysis.

Note. Tolerance may be defined as the need to use larger doses to achieve the same effects with repeated administrations.

33   (a)   True (p. 126): less than 5%.
     (b)   True (p. 126).
     (c)   True (p. 126).
     (d)   True (p. 126).
     (e)   False (p. 126).

Note. A symptom peculiar to benzodiazepine withdrawal is a sensation of abnormal body sway. Of particular note are symptoms of abnormal sensory perception, such as hyperacusis, paraesthesiae, photophobia and hyper-sensitivity to touch and pain and also other somatic symptoms, such as muscle stiffness or twitching.

34   Features of the withdrawal syndrome from benzodiazepines include:
(a)   Symptoms usually emerge during the first week of discontinuation.
(b)   Benzodiazepines with a shorter half-life are more likely to produce symptoms.
(c)   Propranolol decreases the frequency of withdrawal symptoms.
(d)   Usually 4–16 weeks are required in the process of gradual dose reduction.
(e)   Clonidine may reduce the severity of the withdrawal syndrome.

35   The following are correct:
(a)   Propranolol is an antagonist at both beta$_1$ and beta$_2$ adrenoceptors.
(b)   Buspirone is an cyclopyrrolone compound.
(c)   Buspirone is an agonist at 5-HT$_{1A}$ receptors.
(d)   Buspirone can cause an increase in prolactin.
(e)   Buspirone has pro-convulsant effects.

36   The following are tetracyclic antidepressants:
(a)   Maprotiline.
(b)   Viloxazine.
(c)   Bupropion.
(d)   Mianserin.
(e)   Trazodone.

37   The following are true in relation to monoamine oxidase inhibitors (MAOIs):
(a)   Selegiline is a selective MAO-A inhibitor.
(b)   MAOIs' acute neurochemical effects consist of an increase in concentration of noradrenaline and dopamine.
(c)   Prolonged treatment with non-selective MAOIs results in 'down-regulation' of 5-HT$_2$ receptors.
(d)   Tyramine is metabolised by MAO-A in the intestinal mucosa.
(e)   Selective MAO-B inhibitors do not provoke the cheese reaction.

38   The following are properties of MAOIs:
(a)   MAO-B activity can be measured directly.
(b)   Inhibition of MAO-A can be measured directly.
(c)   The non-selective irreversible MAOIs markedly reduce REM sleep.
(d)   Tranylcypromine has some amphetamine-like properties.
(e)   MAOIs increase the concentration of brain 5-HT.

34   (a)  True  (pp. 126–127): persists for 7–10 days. Symptoms of withdrawal also emerge following dose reduction.
  (b)  True  (p. 127): those on drugs with a short half-life should be changed to ones with a longer half-life, from which withdrawal features are less severe.
  (c)  False (p. 127): propranolol attenuates some features but does not decrease the frequency of withdrawal symptoms or improve outcome.
  (d)  True  (p. 127): depending on initial dose.
  (e)  True  (p. 127).

35   (a)  True  (p. 132).
  (b)  False (p. 133): it is an azaspirodecanedione. It does not have affinity for benzodiazepine receptors and does not appear to exert any direct effects on GABA activity. It is thus devoid of anticonvulsant, muscle-relaxant and major sedative effects.
  (c)  True  (p. 133).
  (d)  True  (p. 133): it is an antagonist at presynaptic dopamine receptors but does not antagonise postsynaptic dopamine receptors.
  (e)  True  (p. 134).

36   (a)  True  (p. 140).
  (b)  False (p. 140): it is a bicyclic, as is fluoxetine.
  (c)  False (p. 140): it is a monocyclic, as is fluvoxamine.
  (d)  True  (p. 140).
  (e)  True  (p. 140).

  Note. Tricyclics include imipramine, amitryptyline, dothiepin and amoxepine.

37   (a)  False (p. 143): it is an MAO-B inhibitor. Clorgiline is a selective MAO-A inhibitor.
  (b)  True  (p. 144).
  (c)  True  (p. 144): also 5-HT$_{1A}$.
  (d)  True  (p. 145): also the liver, to a lesser extent.
  (e)  True  (p. 145): but they are ineffective antidepressants.

38   (a)  True  (p. 146): in the platelets.
  (b)  False (p. 146): can be inferred from reductions in the concentration of MHPG in urine and DHPG in plasma.
  (c)  True  (p. 147): results in rebound increase in REM sleep after discontinuation of treatment.
  (d)  True  (p. 147): increase in motor activity and heightened sensitivity to external stimuli. However, there is no tolerance to these effects and the MAOIs cannot substitute for amphetamine in patients addicted to this psychostimulant.
  (e)  True  (p. 144): also increase the concentration of noradrenaline and dopamine.

39　The pharmacokinetics of MAOIs includes:

(a)　Irreversible non-selective MAOIs are highly water soluble.
(b)　They have a short elimination half-life.
(c)　They are mainly excreted unchanged by the kidney.
(d)　About 80% of white people are fast acetylators.
(e)　The acetylation status is polygenically inherited.

40　The following side-effects are noted with MAOIs:

(a)　Insomnia is a frequent complication.
(b)　Paradoxical orthostatic hypotension is one of the most common side-effects.
(c)　Peripheral neuropathy is rare.
(d)　Hepatocellular jaundice is rare.
(e)　Bone marrow suppression is rare.

41　Tricyclic antidepressants have the following properties:

(a)　They inhibit the uptake of noradrenaline and 5-HT into nerve terminals.
(b)　The antimuscarinic action is the basis of many of the peripheral side-effects.
(c)　Tricyclic antidepressants have a moderate affinity for $alpha_2$ adrenoceptors.
(d)　They down-regulate $beta_1$ adrenoceptors.
(e)　Long-term treatment leads to a decreased number of $D_2$ receptors.

42　Tricyclic antidepressants have the following anticholinergic effects:

(a)　Miosis.
(b)　Ejaculatory incompetence.
(c)　Reduced glandular secretion.
(d)　Tachycardia.
(e)　Reduced bowel motility.

43　Tricyclic antidepressants have the following effects on sleep:

(a)　They increase the number of awakenings.
(b)　They decrease the latency to onset of REM sleep.
(c)　Decrease the stage 4 sleep.
(d)　They reduce REM sleep duration.
(e)　They have profound effects on sleep.

39  (a) False (p. 147): they are highly lipid soluble, rapidly absorbed and widely distributed.
    (b) True (p. 147): for example, 1 hour for phenelzine, 2 hours for tranylcypromine.
    (c) False (p. 147): extensively metabolised by the liver. Only 1–2% is excreted unchanged in the urine.
    (d) False (p. 148): 50% of white people and a higher proportion of Orientals are fast acetylators.
    (e) False (p. 147): monogenically inherited acetylator status.

40  (a) True (p. 150): also daytime drowsiness.
    (b) True (p. 151).
    (c) True (p. 151).
    (d) True (p. 152).
    (e) True (p. 152).

    Note. The effects of the MAOIs on the autonomic nervous system are complex: although a sympathomimetic effect predominates, there is also some sympatholytic effect. The sympathomimetic effect can lead to cardiac arrhythmias, tremor and mild 'anticholinergic' side-effects in organs that receive a dual adrenergic/cholinergic innervation.

41  (a) True (p. 156).
    (b) True (p. 157).
    (c) False (p. 157): little affinity for alpha$_2$ adrenoceptors.
    (d) True (p. 157): also 5-HT$_2$ with chronic treatment.
    (e) False (p. 158): D$_1$ dopamine receptors. Long-term treatment also results in increases in GABA$_B$ receptors.

42  (a) False (p. 158): miosis is a sympatholytic effect.
    (b) False (p. 158): ejaculatory incompetence is a sympatholytic effect.
    (c) True (p. 158).
    (d) True (p. 158): it is an anticholinergic effect, and also a sympatho-mimetic effect.
    (e) True (p. 158).

    Note. Anticholinergic effects include reduced glandular secretion, mydriasis, reduced bowel motility, tachycardia, urinary hesitancy and erectile dysfunction. Sympathomimetic effects include tachycardia and mydriasis. Sympatholytic effects include hypotension, miosis and ejaculatory incompetence.

43  (a) False (p. 160): they decrease them.
    (b) False (p. 160): they increase it.
    (c) False (p. 160): they increase it.
    (d) True (p. 160).
    (e) True (p. 160).

44   Tricyclic antidepressants have the following pharmacokinetic properties:

(a)   Amitriptyline delays its own absorption.
(b)   All tricyclic antidepressants are lipid soluble.
(c)   Tricyclic antidepressants are poorly bound to plasma proteins.
(d)   They are extensively metabolised in the liver.
(e)   Smoking may inhibit metabolism via 2-hydroxylation.

45   The following are tricyclic antidepressant side-effects:

(a)   Xerostomia.
(b)   Accommodation block in the eye.
(c)   Decreased myocardial contractility.
(d)   Tachycardia as a consequence of a sympatomimetic effect.
(e)   'Atropine' psychosis.

46   The following drug interactions occur with tricyclic antidepressants:

(a)   Methylphenidate has a hypertensive interaction with tricyclic antidepressants.
(b)   Co-administration with MAOIs can lead to a toxic reaction.
(c)   Tricyclic antidepressants potentiate the pressor effects of directly acting sympatomimetic amines.
(d)   They enhance the antihypertensive effects of adrenergic neuron-blocking agents.
(e)   Butyrophenones enhance the metabolism of tricyclic antidepressants.

47   The following statements regarding tricyclic antidepressant receptor pharmacology are correct:

(a)   Maprotiline is a potent inhibitor of noradrenaline and 5-HT uptake.
(b)   Nomifensine is a selective inhibitor of noradrenaline uptake.
(c)   Reboxetine is a potent and selective inhibitor of noradrenaline uptake with weak anticholinergic properties.
(d)   Viloxazine is a potent inhibitor of dopamine uptake.
(e)   Desipramine blocks noradrenaline and 5-HT uptake.

44   (a)  True (p. 161).
     (b)  True (p. 161): and therefore are almost completely absorbed from
          the gut and rapidly and widely distributed in the tissues of the
          body. They readily cross lipid barriers such as the placenta and the
          blood–brain barrier.
     (c)  False (p. 161): they are extensively bound to plasma proteins (e.g.
          imipramine is 75–95%).
     (d)  True (p. 161).
     (e)  False (p. 161): smoking and barbiturates facilitate and neuroleptics
          inhibit metabolism.

45   (a)  True (p. 165): decreased glandular secretions (anticholinergic effect).
     (b)  True (p. 165): anticholinergic effect.
     (c)  True (p. 166): impaired cardiac conduction is another direct effect.
     (d)  False (p. 166): also as a consequence of anticholinergic effects.
     (e)  True (p. 165): toxic confusional state with potent anticholinergic
          tricyclic antidepressants (e.g. amitriptyline).

46   (a)  True (p. 167).
     (b)  True (p. 167): hyperthermia, mydriasis, hyper-reflexia, convulsions,
          coma.
     (c)  True (p. 167): e.g. adrenaline, noradrenaline, leading to hazardous
          hypertension.
     (d)  False (p. 167): they inhibit the antihypertensive effects, probably
          by blocking the uptake of these drugs into the sympathetic nerve
          terminal (e.g. guanethidine).
     (e)  False (p. 168): they inhibit the metabolism of tricyclic antidepressants.
          Phenothiazines also inhibit their metabolism. Barbiturates facilitate
          their metabolism by the liver, probably by inducing microsomal
          enzymes.

47   (a)  False (p. 169): it has little effect on 5-HT but is a potent inhibitor of
          noradrenaline uptake.
     (b)  False (p. 169): nomifensine blocks noradrenaline uptake. It is also a
          potent inhibitor of dopamine uptake.
     (c)  True (p. 169): it has virtually no affinity for alpha$_1$ adrenoceptors.
     (d)  False (p. 169): viloxazine is a selective but rather weak inhibitor of
          noradrenaline uptake and has only very weak anticholinergic effects.
     (e)  True (p. 169): also blocks muscarinic cholinoceptors, alpha$_1$
          adrenoceptors and H$_1$ histamine receptors.

48 Features of SSRIs include:
(a) Citalopram is the most potent of the SSRIs.
(b) Paroxetine is the most selective.
(c) Fluoxetine is the least potent.
(d) SSRIs suppress REM sleep.
(e) The most common side-effect of a single dose of an SSRI is sleep disturbance.

49 Pharmacokinetic properties of SSRIs include:
(a) Rapid absorption from the gut.
(b) They all have a rather long elimination half-life.
(c) The active metabolite of fluoxetine has an elimination half-life of 6 days.
(d) Fluoxetine requires a 5-week washout prior to administration of an MAOI.
(e) Fluoxetine displays non-linear elimination kinetics.

50 SSRIs have the following effects on the following conditions:
(a) They may reduce both obsessional thinking and compulsive rituals.
(b) They reduce both the frequency and intensity of binges in bulimia nervosa.
(c) They may reduce craving in alcoholic patients.
(d) Fluovoxamine may alleviate the motor stereotypies of Gilles de la Tourette's syndrome.
(e) Cataplexy may benefit from SSRIs.

51 SSRIs have the following drug interactions:
(a) Combination of SSRIs and MAOIs results in the serotonin syndrome.
(b) SSRIs may increase lithium levels.
(c) SSRIs enhance the metabolism of drugs.
(d) Fluvoxamine may increase the clearance of diazepam.
(e) SSRIs increase the levels of tricyclic antidepressants.

48   (a)   False (p. 172): most selective.
     (b)   False (p. 172): most potent.
     (c)   False (p. 172): zimeldine (withdrawn because of toxic reaction, Guillain–Barré syndrome.
     (d)   True (p. 173).
     (e)   False (p. 172): nausea.

     Note. They have little effect on cardiovascular functions, although most SSRIs cause a small drop in heart rate. In general they do not affect autonomic functions.

49   (a)   False (p. 173): slowly but almost completely absorbed from the gut. The time to peak plasma concentration following a single oral dose varies from 2–8 hours (fluvoxamine) to 6–10 hours (sertraline).
     (b)   True (p. 173): which allows once-daily administration. Fluvoxamine has the shortest (15 hours) and fluoxetine the longest (84 hours) plasma half-life.
     (c)   True (p. 174).
     (d)   True (p. 174): because of the slow clearance of fluoxetine and its active metabolite.
     (e)   True (p. 174): probably owing to the saturation of liver enzymes – higher doses can result in disproportionately higher plasma levels.

50   (a)   True (p. 175): the effectiveness of the SSRIs in obsessive–compulsive disorder seems to be independent of their antidepressant activity.
     (b)   True (p. 175): they decrease carbohydrate craving also.
     (c)   True (p. 175): preliminary reports that they can reduce craving and alcohol intake in alcoholic patients.
     (d)   False (p. 175): psychological symptoms of Gilles de la Tourette's syndrome.
     (e)   True (p. 175): some reports that some myoclonic syndromes, cataplexy and chronic pain syndromes may benefit from SSRIs.

51   (a)   True (p. 177): also co-administration of SSRIs with tryptophan or lithium (p. 178) can result in the serotonin syndrome.
     (b)   True (p. 178): also decrease lithium levels.
     (c)   False (p. 178): SSRIs inhibit the metabolism of drugs by the oxidative microsomal enzymes in the liver, and thus can increase the plasma levels of drugs that are metabolised by these enzymes, such as tricyclic antidepressants, warfarin, phenytoin, theophylline, propranolol (but not atenolol).
     (d)   False (p. 178): reduces clearance and thus increases its half-life.
     (e)   True (p. 178): sometimes twofold, as per answer in (c) above.

52 Mianserin:
(a) Inhibits uptake of both noradrenaline and 5-HT.
(b) Has considerable alpha$_1$ adrenoceptor blocking properties.
(c) Has weak antimuscarinic effects.
(d) Has significant sedative effects.
(e) Has a plasma half-life that allows once-daily dosage.

53 Trazodone:
(a) Is a potent inhibitor of 5-HT uptake.
(b) Enhances conditioned avoidance responses.
(c) Its alpha$_1$ adrenoceptor blockage leads to mydriasis.
(d) Can cause orthostatic hypotension.
(e) Follows biphasic elimination kinetics.

54 Common side-effects of mianserin include:
(a) Increased alertness.
(b) Anorexia.
(c) Weight gain.
(d) Hepatocellular jaundice in the young.
(e) Autonomic side-effects in the elderly.

55 The complications of trazadone include:
(a) Nasal congestion.
(b) Ejaculatory incompetence.
(c) Rarely bone marrow suppression.
(d) Contraindication in epilepsy.
(e) Ventricular tachycardia.

52 (a) False (p. 180): it is a potent inhibitor of noradrenaline uptake with little effect on 5-HT or dopamine.
   (b) False (p. 180): it is an alpha$_2$ antagonist and it has weak alpha$_1$ antagonism.
   (c) True (p. 180).
   (d) False (p. 181): it is mildly sedative.
   (e) True (p. 182): it is rapidly absorbed from the gut and the peak plasma concentration appears less than 3 hours after a single oral dose. The plasma half-life is 10–20 hours.

53 (a) False (p. 180): weak inhibition of 5-HT uptake with little affinity for noradrenaline or dopamine. With reference to 5-HT uptake inhibition, it has one-fifteenth the potency of clomipramine.
   (b) False (p. 181): like the antipsychotics, trazodone reduces conditioned avoidance responses without affecting unconditioned responses.
   (c) False (p. 181): miosis and priapism and also hypotension.
   (d) True (p. 181).
   (e) True (p. 182): the half-life of the first phase is 1–4.5 hours and that of the second is 7–13 hours. On multiple dosing the steady-state plasma level is attained within a few days.

54 (a) False (p. 182): drowsiness, which is most marked during the first few weeks of treatment.
   (b) False (p. 182): increased appetite.
   (c) True (p. 182).
   (d) False (p. 182): not common but does occur, especially in elderly.
   (e) False (p. 183): the lack of cardiovascular and autonomic side-effects may benefit some elderly patients, although special caution is needed in this patient group because of the lower rate of elimination and the increased risk of bone marrow and liver damage.

55 (a) True (p. 183): reflects alpha$_1$ adrenoceptor blockade, as does orthostatic hypotension, priapism or ejaculatory incompetence.
   (b) True (p. 183): also priapism.
   (c) True (p. 183): usually mild.
   (d) False (p. 183): special caution is recommended because it possibly decreases seizure threshold. Special caution is also recommended in those with a history of heart disease and hepatic or renal insufficiency.
   (e) True (p. 183): although trazodone shows relatively little cardiotoxicity compared with conventional tricyclic antidepressants, arrhythmias can occur in susceptible patients.

56   Pharmacokinetics of lithium:

(a)   Lithium has a wide therapeutic range.
(b)   It is weakly bound to serum proteins.
(c)   The half-life of lithium lies between 10 and 24 hours.
(d)   It passes freely through the glomerular membrane independent of serum concentration.
(e)   Lithium renal clearance is enhanced with sodium depletion.

57   The following observations contribute to our understanding of lithium's mechanism of action:

(a)   Lithium decreases sodium/potassium adenosine triphosphatase in patients but not controls.
(b)   Short-term lithium treatment decreases brain serotonin turnover in animals.
(c)   The serum cortisol response to 5-hydroxytryptophan is enhanced during lithium treatment.
(d)   Clinical studies suggest a possible lithium-induced reduction in noradrenaline turnover in affective disorders.
(e)   Lithium can block the development of the supersensitivity which develops in dopamine receptors after chronic inhibition by neuroleptics.

58   The following are true of the effects of lithium:

(a)   Approximately 20–40% of patients with mania fail to respond.
(b)   The majority of trials comparing lithium with tricyclic antidepressants show an equivalent response.
(c)   Lithium augmentation of tricyclic antidepressants is believed to act as a combined facilitation of central 5-HT neurotransmission.
(d)   Approximately one-third of those on lithium for recurrent bipolar affective disorder will relapse.
(e)   Combination of lithium and tricyclic antidepressants accords additional benefit in prophylaxis against unipolar depression.

59   Predictors of a good response to lithium include:

(a)   A positive family history of bipolar affective disorder.
(b)   A 'pure' form of bipolar affective disorder.
(c)   Younger age.
(d)   Marital status.
(e)   Depression followed by mania.

56   (a)   False (p.194): it has a narrow therapeutic range, that is, compared with other drugs, there is a narrow gap between the minimum blood level (0.4 mmol/l) required for therapeutic efficacy and the maximum level (1.5 mmol/l), beyond which toxicity may ensue.
　　　(b)   False (p. 194): it is not bound.
　　　(c)   True (p. 194).
　　　(d)   True (p. 195).
　　　(e)   False (p. 194): lithium renal clearance is reduced when sodium is depleted, reduced intake or excess loss thus risking toxic serum levels of lithium.

57   (a)   False (p. 196): it increases sodium/potassium ATPase in patients but not controls.
　　　(b)   False (p. 196): it increases it.
　　　(c)   True (p. 196): also true for prolactin response to tryptophan.
　　　(d)   True (p. 197).
　　　(e)   True (p. 197).

58   (a)   True (p. 198).
　　　(b)   True (p. 199).
　　　(c)   True (p. 200).
　　　(d)   True (p. 200): compared with 80% of those on placebo.
　　　(e)   False (p. 201): no additional benefit. Although lithium is the drug of first choice in the prophylaxis of bipolar affective disorder, it is the second choice in unipolar disorders, next to SSRIs.

59   (a)   True (p. 202).
　　　(b)   True (p. 202).
　　　(c)   False (p. 202): age is not a predictor.
　　　(d)   False (p. 202): marital status is not a predictor.
　　　(e)   False (p. 202): episodic sequence of mania followed by depression.

Note. Predictors of a positive response include: patient compliance, a good previous response, a 'pure' form of bipolar affective illness or endogenous type of depression, a family history of bipolar illness, an episodic sequence of mania followed by depression rather than depression followed by mania. Low neuroticism and high obsessionality may predict a good outcome. Predictors of a poor response include: rapid cycling, paranoid features, substance misuse, poor social support, living with relatives rated as being of high expressed emotion. Factors which are not predictors include: age, marital status, response to dexamethasone suppression test, thyroid and renal function.

60 Signs of lithium intoxication include:
(a) Fine tremor.
(b) Increased viscosity of pulmonary secretions.
(c) Diarrhoea.
(d) Dysphasia.
(e) Decreased motoric activity.

61 The following effects occur in more than one-third of patients treated with lithium:
(a) Memory problems.
(b) Weight gain.
(c) Drowsiness.
(d) T-wave flattening and inversion.
(e) Metallic taste.

62 Lithium has the following effects on the kidney:
(a) 30% of patients show histological abnormalities.
(b) Lithium inhibits the antidiuretic hormone (ADH) response to cAMP.
(c) Lithium has a significant effect on glomeral filtration rate (GFR).
(d) Discontinuation of lithium invariably leads to reversal of polyuria.
(e) Once-daily dosage is probably safer for the kidney.

63 The following are true statements with regard to the administration of lithium during pregnancy:
(a) The risk of Epstein's anomaly is 1%.
(b) Foetal goitre can complicate delivery.
(c) Lithium dosage generally requires reduction in pregnancy.
(d) Lithium concentrations in breast milk are 90% of maternal serum concentrations.
(e) The first trimester is an absolute contraindication to lithium therapy.

60   (a)  False (p. 205): coarse tremor.
     (b)  True (p. 205).
     (c)  True (p. 205).
     (d)  False (p. 205): dysarthria.
     (e)  False (p. 205): restlessness.

     Note. Additional signs include vomiting, ataxia, cognitive impairment, lassitude, restlessness, agitation. Seizures and coma may follow. Death is as a result of either cardiac effects or pulmonary complications caused by severe viscosity of respiratory secretions. The signs may appear at serum levels above 1.3 mmol/l. Treatment involves supportive measures, anti-epileptics when indicated and increase in fluid intake (sometimes saline infusion) and haemodialysis when the serum level is above 3 mmol/l, there is coma or shock or where conservative measures have failed.

61   (a)  True (p. 206): reported as high as 52% in one study.
     (b)  False (p. 206): approximately 20%.
     (c)  False (p. 206): approximately 25%.
     (d)  False (p. 209): up to 30%.
     (e)  False (p. 206): infrequent complaint, as is a complaint of altered psychosexual problems.

     Note. Other such effects include polyuria (approximately 40%) and tremor (approximately 35%).

62   (a)  False (p. 206): approximately 10–15%.
     (b)  False (p. 207): inhibits cAMP response to ADH in the cells of the collecting ducts.
     (c)  False (p. 207): a modest effect on the GFR as measured by creatinine clearance.
     (d)  False (p. 207): often but not invariably.
     (e)  True (p. 207): based on experimental work in rats.

63   (a)  False (p. 210): 0.1%, although this is still 20 times greater than that in the normal population.
     (b)  True (p. 210): foetal goitre presses on the trachea.
     (c)  False (p. 210): lithium dosage will require compensatory increases because GFR improves gradually.
     (d)  False (p. 210): concentrations in breast milk are 50% of the maternal serum concentration, although infants may have similar blood levels, as their capacity to handle lithium is less. Breast-feeding is therefore relatively contraindicated.
     (e)  False (p. 210): risk–benefit analysis is required, in which the risks to mother and foetus of not taking lithium need to be considered.

64   The following are true of carbamazepine:

(a)   Teratogenically, there is an increased risk of spina bifida.
(b)   It may induce its own metabolism.
(c)   When leucopenia results carbamazepine should be automatically discontinued.
(d)   There are strong positive correlations between blood levels and side-effects.
(e)   Should not be combined with MAOIs.

65   Common side-effects of valproate include:

(a)   Thrombocytopenia.
(b)   Cognitive dysfunction.
(c)   Ankle swelling.
(d)   Hair thinning.
(e)   Hepatotoxicity.

66   The following are haematological effects of carbamazepine:

(a)   Leucopenia.
(b)   Hyponatraemia.
(c)   Leucocytosis.
(d)   Agranulocytosis.
(e)   Aplastic anaemia.

67   Biochemical effects of electroconvulsive therapy (ECT) include:

(a)   Plasma noradrenaline rises acutely.
(b)   Plasma concentration of 5-HIAA rises acutely.
(c)   Prolactin elevation is the most common acute hormonal change.
(d)   Dopamine does not appear to be affected.
(e)   Plasma levels of adrenocorticotrophin-releasing hormone (ACTH) are elevated.

64  (a)  True (p. 216): there appears to be an increase in developmental disorders such as spina bifida in children born to epileptic mothers on carbamazepine.
    (b)  True (p. 216): blood levels may therefore drop. Likewise it may reduce blood levels of other drugs, including antipsychotics.
    (c)  False (p. 216): not if asymptomatic or non-progressive leucopenia develops. If it is severe, progressive or produces clinical symptoms such as sore throat, then carbamazepine should be stopped.
    (d)  False (p. 216): nor is there a positive correlation with clinical benefits.
    (e)  True (p. 216): because of its structural similarity to tricyclic antidepressants.

65  (a)  False (p. 217): less common.
    (b)  True (p. 217).
    (c)  True (p. 217).
    (d)  True (p. 217).
    (e)  False (p. 217): less common.

      Note. Common side-effects include: tremor, weight gain, ankle swelling, hair thinning, cognitive dysfunction. Less common side-effects include: hepatotoxicity, thrombocytopenia, metabolic abnormality (hyperammonaemia/glycinaemia), encephalopathy, toxicity (1–2%).

66  (a)  True (p. 215).
    (b)  False (p. 215): it is a metabolic effect.
    (c)  False (p. 215).
    (d)  True (p. 215).
    (e)  True (p. 215).

      Note. A full blood count should be carried out before treatment, weekly for the first month, monthly for the subsequent five months; and two to four times a year thereafter. Carbamazepine does not have to be automatically stopped if an asymptomatic or non-progressive leucopenia develops.

67  (a)  True (p. 236): for up to 5 minutes with each ECT treatment.
    (b)  False (p. 237): not altered acutely, but 24-hour urinary 5-HIAA excretion may fall.
    (c)  True (p. 237): prolactin is stimulated by 5-HT and inhibited by dopamine inputs. The prolactin surge with ECT is probably linked to stimulation of the 5-HT$_1$ receptor subtype.
    (d)  False (p. 238): appears to affect dopamine systems but exact nature is unclear.
    (e)  True (p. 238): by each ECT treatment. Plasma cortisol rises acutely between 5 and 15 minutes after ECT and remains elevated for at least 60 minutes. The rise in plasma cortisol is most pronounced in non-psychotic depression.

      Note. Box 7.1 on p. 240 gives a useful summary of the acute hormonal changes with ECT and Box 7.2 on p. 241 gives a useful summary of the hormonal changes with ECT over the course of treatment.

68  The following are acute increased hormonal changes with ECT:
(a)  Thyroid-stimulating hormone (TSH).
(b)  Neurophysins.
(c)  Vasopressin.
(d)  Substance P.
(e)  Insulin.

69  Plausible explanations of the therapeutic effects of ECT are supported by the following:
(a)  Reduction of plasma concentration of noradrenaline.
(b)  Decrease in dopamine function.
(c)  Increase of 5-HT function.
(d)  Increase of corticotrophin-releasing hormone (CRH) concentration in cerebrospinal fluid (CSF).
(e)  A blunting of TSH response to thyrotrophin-releasing hormone (TRH).

70  The following are true in relation to seizure and efficacy:
(a)  Bilateral ECT is many times more effective than unilateral ECT.
(b)  The magnitude of the stimulus has a strong relationship to side-effects.
(c)  The magnitude of the stimulus has a strong relationship to seizure threshold.
(d)  Seizure time has a strong relationship to efficacy.
(e)  Seizure threshold rises and seizure duration shortens in the course of a typical series of treatments.

71  The following side-effects of ECT affect approximately 10% of patients:
(a)  Headache.
(b)  Palpitations.
(c)  Confusion.
(d)  Drowsiness.
(e)  Weakness.

72  ECT and memory:
(a)  Memory impairment is associated with the amount of electrical energy.
(b)  Unilateral ECT applied to the dominant hemisphere appears to induce less memory impairment.
(c)  Short-term retrograde amnesia may extend back for a few weeks.
(d)  Memory impairment generally resolves within 3 months.
(e)  Short-term anterograde amnesia is more severe with bilateral ECT.

68   (a)  True (p. 240): also cortisol, prolactin, ACTH, beta-endorphin, oxytocin.
     (b)  True (p. 240).
     (c)  True (p. 240).
     (d)  True (p. 240).
     (e)  True (p. 240).

69   (a)  True (p. 242).
     (b)  False (p. 242): an increase in dopamine function.
     (c)  True (p. 242).
     (d)  False (p. 242): a decrease of CRH concentration in CSF.
     (e)  False (p. 241): no blunting. Baseline TRH and TSH are unaltered by a course of ECT. Free thyroxine appears to fall with ECT in a manner unrelated to clinical improvement, plasma albumin or fatty acid concentrations.

70   (a)  True (p. 243).
     (b)  False (p. 243): little relationship.
     (c)  True (p. 243).
     (d)  False (p. 244): little relationship to efficacy; however, very short seizures (less than 20 seconds) are likely to be the result of inadequate stimulus in relation to a patient's seizure threshold.
     (e)  True (p. 244).

71   (a)  False (p. 245): 30%, and more commonly after bilateral than after unilateral ECT.
     (b)  True (p. 245).
     (c)  True (p. 245).
     (d)  True (p. 245).
     (e)  True (p. 245).
          Note. Additionally, muscular pains and hypotension.

72   (a)  True (p. 246): appears to be so, and also to the site of the electrodes.
     (b)  False (p. 247): non-dominant hemisphere but this also appears to be less clinically effective.
     (c)  True (p. 247): genearlly, for a few hours to a few days before treatment. This impairment can be caused by both ECT and the depressive illness.
     (d)  False (p. 247): over 6 months.
     (e)  True (p. 247): this is more common and affects the ability to learn new information. It resolves rapidly and usually completely by 6 months.

73   Features accepted to predict a good response to ECT include:
(a)   Psychomotor retardation.
(b)   Somatic delusions.
(c)   Weight loss.
(d)   Feeling worse in the evening.
(e)   Hypochondriasis.

74   The following are true of dopamine receptor subtypes:
(a)   $D_1$ increases cAMP.
(b)   $D_1$ is concentrated in the hippocampus.
(c)   $D_4$ is relatively localised to mesolimbic and mesocortical tracts.
(d)   $D_3$ receptor has a distinct regional localisation in the limbic system.
(e)   Clozapine has a tenfold higher affinity for $D_4$ than for $D_2$ receptors.

75   The following are true of clozapine:
(a)   The incidence of agranulocytosis is 2–3%.
(b)   Approximately one-third of treatment-resistant patients respond within 6 weeks of treatment.
(c)   Sialorrhoea is a common side-effect.
(d)   Where combination with an anticonvulsant is required sodium valproate should be avoided.
(e)   Severe rebound psychosis may occur within a week on abrupt discontinuation.

76   Objections to the dopamine hypothesis of schizophrenia are supported by the following:
(a)   A decrease in $D_2$ receptor population in post-mortem brain in schizophrenia.
(b)   Serum prolactin is not decreased in untreated schizophrenia.
(c)   Poor correlation between dopamine blockade and clinical response.
(d)   Negative symptoms are minimally improved with dopamine blockade.
(e)   Positron emission tomography (PET) scan studies of dopamine receptors in the brain of schizophrenic patients failed to show any difference between untreated patients and 'normal' controls.

73  (a) True (p. 249): although this feature also predicted a good response to simulated ECT in the Northwick Park ECT trial (1984).
    (b) True (p. 248).
    (c) True (p. 248).
    (d) False (p. 248).
    (e) False (p. 248).

    Note. The prognostic value of some features has not been widely replicated. There seems, however, to be a consensus regarding delusions, psychomotor retardation and 'endogenous' depression as predictors of a good response to ECT. Indicators of a poor response to ECT seem to be the presence of recent precipitants to the illness and personality factors.

74  (a) True (p. 267): as does $D_5$.
    (b) False (p. 267): $D_1$ receptors are found in the caudate, putamen, nucleus accumbens and olfactory tubercle. $D_5$ is found in the hippocampus and hypothalamus.
    (c) True (pp. 267, 268): it is found in the mesolimbic and mesocortical tracts and medulla, midbrain and frontal cortex.
    (d) True (pp. 267, 268): $D_3$ is localised in the limbic system (olfactory tubercle, hypothalamus and nucleus accumbens).
    (e) True (p. 268).

    Note. $D_2$ receptors decrease cAMP and are concentrated in the caudate, putamen, nucleus accumbens and olfactory tubercle.

75  (a) True (p. 271).
    (b) True (p. 271): a further one-third will respond within one year.
    (c) True (p. 300): particularly at night.
    (d) False (p. 301): carbamazepine should be avoided and sodium valproate is preferable.
    (e) True (p. 301): in approximately half of the patients who discontinue it abruptly.

76  (a) False (p. 275): actually an increase in $D_2$ receptors in post-mortem brain in schizophrenia is found, which is supportive evidence of the dopamine hypothesis.
    (b) True (p. 275).
    (c) True (p. 275).
    (d) True (p. 275).
    (e) True (p. 275).

    Note. Further objections to the dopamine hypothesis are: homovanillic acid (HVA) is not usually elevated in the CSF; psychotic symptoms are not closely or invariably associated with any other evidence of increased dopamine receptor sensitivity; and there is a time lag of 3–4 weeks before the onset of the therapeutic effect after dopamine blockade.

77 The following are true regarding neuroleptics and their effects on cognition:
(a) Chronic treatment does not cause any significant impairment on psychometric tests.
(b) Impairments in memory could be attributed to nigrostriatal dopamine blockade.
(c) Impairments of fine motor coordination can be attributed to antimuscarinic effects of neuroleptics.
(d) Chronic treatment is associated with improvements on most measures of cognition and attention.
(e) Impairments in cognitive and psychomotor functions occur after acute treatment in normal healthy volunteers but not patients.

78 The endocrine effects of neuroleptics include:
(a) False pregnancy test.
(b) Weight gain.
(c) Lactorrhoea.
(d) Primary amenorrhoea.
(e) Unilateral gynaecomastia.

79 Akathisia:
(a) Occurs in up to 50% of patients.
(b) Is characterised by dysphoria.
(c) Acute forms are related to rapid increases in neuroleptic dose.
(d) Chronic forms respond well to anticholinergics.
(e) Is synonymous with the restless legs syndrome.

80 Correct statements regarding tardive dyskinesia include:
(a) Incidence of approximately 15%.
(b) Hemiballismus is not a feature.
(c) Involvement of mouth and face is rare in children.
(d) It may be made worse by anticholinergic medication.
(e) It is likely that a combination of anticholinergic and neuroleptic drugs is associated with an increased prevalence.

77   (a)  True (p. 276): nor psychomotor performance.
     (b)  False (p. 276): antimuscarinic effects of neuroleptics.
     (c)  False (p. 276): nigrostriatal dopamine blockade.
     (d)  True (p. 276): which parallels patients' clinical recovery.
     (e)  False (p. 276): both patients and normal healthy volunteers.

78   (a)  True (p. 281).
     (b)  True (p. 281).
     (c)  True (p. 281).
     (d)  False (p. 281): secondary.
     (e)  True (p. 281).

       Note. The endocrine effects are relatively uncommon and are probably
       largely due to elevated prolactin, whose release is normally inhibited by
       dopamine. In addition to the above side-effects, there may be impotence.

79   (a)  True (p. 285): it may occur to some extent in up to 50%.
     (b)  True (p. 285): characteristics include motor restlessness, subjective
          agitation and dysphoria or intolerance of activity. Dysphoria may
          be an early prodrome of akathisia.
     (c)  True (p. 286).
     (d)  False (p. 286): poorly; may respond better to benzodiazepines.
     (e)  False (p. 286): idiopathic 'restless legs syndrome' is not associated
          with neuroleptics but interestingly often responds to levo-dopa.

       Note. The underlying mechanism of akathisia is unclear and the response
       to anticholinergic treatment is variable. Acute forms are related to rapid
       increases in neuroleptic dose and may respond to anticholinergics. Chronic
       forms may be exacerbated by neuroleptic withdrawal, respond poorly to
       anticholinergics but may respond to benzodiazepines. The best established
       treatment is propranolol.

80   (a)  True (p. 286): although the reported incidence has been as high as
          56%, the overall mean is probably about 15%.
     (b)  False (p. 286): hemiballismus can occur. In addition, orofacial and
          buccal-lingual involuntary movements, choreoathetoid movements
          of upper and lower limbs, a range of tics, abnormal postures, grunting
          vocalisations and disturbances of respiration.
     (c)  True (p. 286): the more peripheral manifestations usually occur in
          patients under 50 years of age.
     (d)  True (p. 286): it may be precipitated by anticholinergic medication
          in some cases.
     (e)  False (p. 286): there is no evidence despite the belief.

81   The following are allergic reactions to neuroleptics:
(a)   Contact dermatitis.
(b)   Stellate opacities in the lens.
(c)   Cholestatic jaundice.
(d)   Optic neuritis.
(e)   Aplastic anaemia.

82   True statements regarding the pharmacokinetics of neuroleptics include:
(a)   PET studies have shown 40% occupancy of brain $D_2$ receptors after normal neuroleptic doses.
(b)   Intramuscular doses of chlorpromazine lead to twofold higher serum levels than corresponding oral doses.
(c)   About 40% of non-responders are poor absorbers of oral chlorpromazine.
(d)   Plasma neuroleptic levels correlate with prolactin increases.
(e)   Haloperidol has a high therapeutic index.

83   Pharmacodynamic interactions:
(a)   Phenothiazines potentiate the central depressant actions of antihistamines.
(b)   Phenothiazines decrease the analgesic effects of opiates.
(c)   Phenothiazines potentiate the central depressant effect of general anaesthetics.
(d)   Butyrophenones cause a marked increase in intracellular lithium.
(e)   Neuroleptics enhance the dopaminergic effects of anti-Parkinsonian drugs.

81 (a) True (p. 292): also an urticarial rash (hypersensitivity), photo-sensitivity and abnormal pigmentation.

(b) True (p. 292): stellate opacities in the anterior part of the lens, the cornea, sclera or conjunctiva); pigmentary retinopathy also (which is dose dependent and occurs notably after high doses of thioridazine).

(d) True (p. 292).

(e) True (p. 292): also agranulocytosis (incidence of 1 in 1300 has been reported).

Note. The precise mechanisms for these reactions are not known, and both allergic and idiosyncratic reactions may be involved in the adverse effects on the eye and the blood.

82 (a) False (p. 295): 65–90% occupancy of brain $D_2$ receptors. Similar occupancies have been found in treatment-resistant patients. It appears that receptor occupancy above 70% is a necessary but not sufficient requirement for an antipsychotic response.

(b) False (p. 294): fourfold or even higher serum levels than the corresponding oral dose because chlorpromazine is highly protein bound, is almost entirely metabolised, undergoes extensive first-pass metabolism and gives rise to at least 150 metabolites, several of which are active.

(c) True (p. 294): because of its metabolism to inactive substances in the intestinal wall (active metabolites being formed in the liver).

(d) True (p. 294): neuroleptic levels also correlate with adverse effects, some EEG changes (increases in delta and theta activity and a decrease in fast beta activity), but not correlate with clinical response.

(e) False (p. 295): it has a low therapeutic index, that is the dose at which first signs of extrapyramidal signs (EPS) occur appears to be very close to the dose required for an optimum antipsychotic effect in most patients.

83 (a) True (p. 296): also true for alcohol and benzodiazepines.

(b) False (p. 296): they cause an increase in the analgesic effects.

(c) True (p. 296): also true for hypotensive effects of general anaesthetics.

(d) False (p. 297): they can cause a minor increase in intracellular lithium.

(e) False (p. 297): they antagonise the dopaminergic effects of anti-Parkinsonian drugs.

84   The following are true of neuroleptics:
(a)   Tolerance to the antipsychotic effect of chlorpromazine does not occur.
(b)   The combination of clozapine and phenytoin should be avoided.
(c)   Haloperidol is non-sedative.
(d)   Risperidone has combined $D_1$ and 5-$HT_2$ antagonistic properties.
(e)   Sulpiride has a high affinity for the tuberoinfundibular tract.

85   Epidemiology of epilepsy:
(a)   1 in 20 people in the general population will have had an epileptic seizure.
(b)   It is commoner in females.
(c)   It is evenly distributed throughout socio-economic groups.
(d)   About 50% of people with epilepsy have no evidence of an underlying structural lesion.
(e)   Reflex epilepsies occur in 10% of people with epilepsy.

86   Precipitating factors of epilepsy in susceptible people include:
(a)   Hyperglycaemia.
(b)   Hypersomnia.
(c)   Hypothermia.
(d)   Hypoventilation.
(e)   Hypoxia.

87   Phenytoin:
(a)   Follows first-order kinetics.
(b)   Is a potent enzyme inhibitor.
(c)   The serum concentration can fall precipitously following a modest dose reduction.
(d)   At around 40 µmol/l neurotoxic symptoms become increasingly likely.
(e)   Causes facial coarsening.

84  (a)  True  (p. 300): but it does to the sedative effect.
    (b)  False (p. 301): where combination with an anticonvulsant is required, sodium valproate is preferable and carbamazepines should be avoided.
    (c)  True (p. 302): it is also free of hypotensive and anticholinergic adverse effects. However, EPS are much commoner and more severe than with chlorpromazine.
    (d)  False (p. 304): $D_2$ and $5\text{-}HT_2$ antagonist. It also has noradrenergic- and histamine-blocking actions but no anticholinergic effects.
    (e)  True  (p. 305): causes galactorrhoea. It has a low incidence of EPS and tardive dyskinesia; it is non-sedative.

85  (a)  True  (p. 332): at some time in their lives, and 1 in 200 will have epilepsy (recurring seizures).
    (b)  False (p. 332): slightly more common in males.
    (c)  False (p. 332): higher in lower socio-economic groups.
    (d)  False (p. 333): approximately 75%.
    (e)  False (p. 334): 1–6%, that is, fits occurring as a direct reflex response to a specific stimulus.

86  (a)  False (p. 334): hypoglycaemia.
    (b)  False (p. 334): sleep deprivation.
    (c)  False (p. 334): hyperpyrexia.
    (d)  False (p. 334): hyperventilation.
    (e)  True  (p. 334).

    Note. A number of precipitating factors may provoke a fit in susceptible people or exacerbate established epilepsy; in addition to the above are anti-depressant and neuroleptic drugs, alcohol and drug withdrawal and the stimuli of reflex epilepsy.

87  (a)  False (p. 342): zero-order kinetics at therapeutic doses. As the concentration rises, the capacity of the hepatic mono-oxygenase enzyme system to metabolise the drug becomes saturated. When this occurs a small increment in dose can result in a large rise in serum levels. Conversely, the serum concentration can fall precipitously following a modest dose reduction.
    (b)  False (p. 342): potent enzyme inducer.
    (c)  True  (p. 342).
    (d)  False (p. 342): over 80 µmol/l.
    (e)  True  (p. 342): also acne, hirsutism, gum hyperplasia.

88 Vigabatrin:

(a) Is a gamma-amino acid.
(b) Is a reversible inhibitor of GABA transaminase.
(c) Is extensively metabolised by the liver.
(d) Has somnolence as a common side-effect.
(e) Can increase plasma phenytoin levels.

89 The following statements are true for lamotrigine:

(a) It enhances the release of excitatory amino acids.
(b) Its pharmacokinetics are linear.
(c) It is a strong hepatic enzyme inducer.
(d) It is an adjunctive therapy for treatment of refractory partial seizures.
(e) Skin rashes occur in 10% of patients.

90 The following are true for gabapentin.

(a) Freely crosses the blood–brain barrier.
(b) Is well tolerated and causes no drug interactions.
(c) Acts pharmacologically as a GABA mimetic.
(d) Is excreted unchanged in the urine.
(e) Peak anticonvulsant action is delayed despite early peak concentration following administration.

91 The following are well-recognised side-effects of carbamazepine.

(a) Peripheral oedema.
(b) Tremor.
(c) Hypoglycaemia.
(d) Psychosis.
(e) Megaloblastic anaemia.

88   (a)   True  (p. 345): with a structure similar to GABA.
     (b)   False (p. 345): irreversible.
     (c)   False (p. 345): not metabolised by liver and not plasma bound, hence
           there is little interaction with other drugs. However, it does cause a
           fall in phenytoin levels by an unknown mechanism.
     (d)   True  (p. 345): tends to remit with continued exposure to the drug.
           Fatigue is also relatively common.
     (e)   False (p. 345): decreased by 20–30%.

89   (a)   False (p. 345): inhibits the release of excitatory amino acids, especially
           glutamate from presynaptic terminals.
     (b)   True  (p. 346).
     (c)   False (p. 346): no effect.
     (d)   True  (p. 345).
     (e)   True  (p. 346): erythema multiforme or maculopapular type.

90   (a)   True  (p. 346): even though it is hydrophilic. It is related in structure
           to GABA.
     (b)   True  (p. 346): no drug interactions have been reported.
     (c)   False (p. 346): despite being structurally similar to GABA.
     (d)   True  (p. 346).
     (e)   True  (p. 348): the concentration of gabapentin in brain interstitial
           space peaks soon after administration; the time of peak anti-
           convulsant action is delayed and occurs as the gabapentin levels
           in the extracellular space in the brain are already starting to decline.

91   (a)   False (p. 349): recognised side-effect of sodium valproate. It is a rare
           side-effect with carbamazepine.
     (b)   False (p. 349): side-effect of sodium valproate.
     (c)   False (p. 349): side-effect of phenytoin.
     (d)   False (p. 349): side-effect of ethosuximide.
     (e)   False (p. 349): side-effect of phenytoin.

      Note. Predictable side-effects of carbamazepine include: diplopia, dizziness,
      drowsiness, headache, nausea, hypernatraemia, hypocalcaemia, orofacial
      dyskinesia, cardiac arrhythmia. Idiosyncratic reactions include: agranulocytosis,
      aplastic anaemia, hepatotoxicity, photosensitivity, Stevens–Johnson syndrome,
      lupus-like syndrome, morbilliform rash, thrombocytopenia, pseudolymphoma.

92 Potent enzyme inducers include:
(a) Phenytoin.
(b) Primidone.
(c) Phenobarbitone.
(d) Carbamazepine.
(e) Sodium valproate.

93 The following statements are true:
(a) Phenytoin therapy should be avoided in young people.
(b) Sodium valproate may be displaced by phenytoin.
(c) Phenytoin is associated with pseudodementia.
(d) Oral contraceptive failure is most likely with sodium valproate.
(e) Carbamazepine is relatively safe in pregnancy.

94 Features of foetal hydantoin syndrome include:
(a) Retarded growth.
(b) Hypertelorism.
(c) Narrow mouth.
(d) Epicanthic folds.
(e) Low-set ears.

95 Conduct disorders in childhood predict the following outcomes in later life:
(a) Poor marital adjustment.
(b) Deficient parenting skills.
(c) Higher rates of premature death.
(d) Poor employment histories.
(e) Increases in psychiatric disorders.

92  (a)  True  (p. 350).
    (b)  True  (p. 350).
    (c)  True  (p. 350).
    (d)  True  (p. 350).
    (e)  False (p. 350): inhibits breakdown of carbamazepine, phenytoin, phenobarbitone and ethosuximide.

> Note. Liver enzyme induction can increase the rate of metabolism of many drugs, resulting in lower plasma levels and so lessened efficacy. Phenytoin, phenobarbitone, primidone and carbamazepine are potent enzyme inducers that tend to lower the plasma levels of each other and of other drugs, such as sodium valproate and the benzodiazepines. Enzyme inhibitors include: cimetidine, erythromycin, isoniazid, verapamil, viloxazine, dextropropoxyphene, danazol, diltiazem, aminodarone, sodium valproate, allpurinol, chloramphenicol, imipramine, metronidazole, phenothiazines and sulphonamides.

93  (a)  True  (p. 342): because of the difficulties caused by its saturable metabolism and the array of cosmetic effects (gum hyperplasia, acne, hirsutism and facial coarsening). Similarly for females of any age.
    (b)  False (p. 350): the reverse is true.
    (c)  True  (p. 352): especially in younger patients with mental handicaps. This is usually associated with toxic serum concentrations of the drug.
    (d)  False (p. 359): sodium is a liver enzyme inhibitor. Failure of oral contraceptives is most likely with inducers, such as phenytoin, phenobarbitone, primidone and carbamazepine.
    (e)  True  (p. 353): sodium valproate has been associated with a high incidence of spina bifida abnormalities. Phenytoin has been associated with the foetal hydantoin syndrome. Cleft lip and palate and cardiovascular abnormalities are known to occur with sodium valproate, phenytoin, phenobarbitone, primidone and trimethadione.

94  (a)  True  (p. 353): also mental retardation, associated with phenytoin.
    (b)  True  (p. 353).
    (c)  False (p. 353): widened mouth and flattened bridge of nose.
    (d)  True  (p. 353).
    (e)  True  (p. 353).

95  (a)  True  (p. 375).
    (b)  True  (p. 375).
    (c)  True  (pp. 375–376).
    (d)  True  (p. 375).
    (e)  True  (p. 375).

96   Tolerance develops to the following drugs:
(a)   Opioids.
(b)   Cocaine.
(c)   Amphetamines.
(d)   Alprazolam.
(e)   Ethanol.

97   The following are true in relation to physical dependence on opioids:
(a)   There is a marked increase in the number of opioid receptors following chronic administration.
(b)   There is a decrease in the functional activity of opioid receptors following chronic administration.
(c)   There is an increase in adenylate cyclase activity.
(d)   There is excessive parasympathetic activity associated with abrupt withdrawal.
(e)   Clonidine acts on mu receptors and attenuates withdrawal symptoms.

98   Pharmacokinetics of alcohol:
(a)   Approximately 75% of alcohol is oxidised in the liver.
(b)   Oxidation is not influenced by the individual's tolerance.
(c)   Elimination follows linear kinetics.
(d)   Metabolic tolerance develops at a slower rate than psychological tolerance.
(e)   'Reverse tolerance' is common.

99   Alcohol:
(a)   Selectively inhibits monoamine oxidase-A.
(b)   Selectively inhibits sodium/potassium-dependent ATP.
(c)   Decreases adenylate cyclase activity.
(d)   Facilitates central inhibitory transmission.
(e)   There is evidence of increased GABA-benzodiazepine receptor function following chronic alcohol administration.

96  (a)  True  (p. 413).
    (b)  False  (p. 414).
    (c)  False  (p. 414).
    (d)  True  (p. 413).
    (e)  True  (p. 413).

> Note. Tolerance means an increasing amount of the drug must be administered to obtain the required pharmacological effect. It may occur as a result of the drug being more rapidly metabolised, so-called metabolic tolerance, or through a drug-induced insensitivity of the receptors or target sites upon which it acts within the brain, termed tissue tolerance (e.g. with anticholinergic agents and sedatives of the benzodiazepine type).

97  (a)  False  (p. 415): no significant change.
    (b)  True  (p. 415).
    (c)  False  (p. 415): a decrease in adenylate cyclase activity, indicative of a decrease in the functional activity of opiod receptors.
    (d)  False  (p. 415): excessive sympathetic activity associated with abrupt withdrawal.
    (e)  False  (p. 415): clonidine acts on $alpha_2$ adrenoceptors; opiates act on mu and delta receptors.

98  (a)  False  (p. 416): over 90% (to carbon dioxide and water).
    (b)  False  (p. 416): oxidation is dependent on the degree of tolerance. The non-tolerant person oxidises at a rate of 10–15 ml of absolute alcohol per hour.
    (c)  False  (p. 416): alcohol follows zero-order kinetics.
    (d)  True  (p. 417).
    (e)  False  (p. 417): reverse tolerance to alcohol, whereby an alcoholic taking a small amount of alcohol becomes intoxicated, aggressive and antisocial, has been described. Cross-tolerance also readily occurs between alcohol and other central depressants (e.g. benzodiazepines and barbiturates).

99  (a)  False  (p. 417): only monoamine oxidase-B.
    (b)  True  (p. 417): in the neuronal membrane but not glial membrane.
    (c)  False  (p. 417): increases.
    (d)  True  (p. 418): it has pronounced sedative properties.
    (e)  False  (p. 418): decreased function, which may be causally related to dependence.

100 The following are true:

(a) Analgesia principally involves the activation of delta receptors.
(b) Naloxone is antagonistic at kappa receptors.
(c) Kappa agonists produce dysphoria.
(d) Opioid analgesics alter the perception of pain.
(e) Opiates cause constipation by inducing spasm of the stomach and intestines.

101 The following occur subsequent to the sudden reduction in plasma opiate levels:

(a) Joint pains.
(b) Miosis.
(c) Piloerection.
(d) Hypothermia.
(e) Anhidrosis.

102 Cocaine:

(a) Cocaine is a major alkaloid from *Papaver coca*.
(b) 'Crack' refers to smoking the free alkaloid.
(c) Cocaine has a half-life of 4 hours.
(d) 50% of users become psychologically dependent.
(e) Cardiovascular complications are the most serious toxic effects.

103 LSD:

(a) LSD is an antagonist at presynaptic 5-HT receptors in the brain.
(b) LSD produces peripheral sympathomimetic effects.
(c) Synaesthesia has been described.
(d) Tolerance can occur after 3 or 4 daily doses.
(e) Anxiety is the commonest feature of abrupt withdrawal.

104 The following are true of phencyclidine (PCP):

(a) It has stimulant and depressant properties.
(b) Small doses produce signs of intoxication.
(c) Higher doses cause catatonic rigidity.
(d) It is a potent amnestic agent.
(e) It exhibits a neuroprotective effect against nerve cell damage arising from cerebral hypoxia.

100 (a) False (p. 423): mu, kappa and delta to a lesser extent.
    (b) True (p. 423): also mu and delta.
    (c) True (p. 424): morphine produces euphoria.
    (d) False (pp. 424–425): opiates attenuate the affective reaction to pain without affecting the perception of pain. Non-opioid analgesics reduce the perception of peripherally mediated pain, by reducing the synthesis of local hormones that activate pain fibres.
    (e) True (p. 426): presumed by stimulation of opioid receptor in the myenteric plexus.

101 (a) True (p. 427).
    (b) False (p. 427): mydriasis.
    (c) True (p. 427).
    (d) False (p. 427): fever.
    (e) False (p. 427): perspiration.

    Note. In addition, restlessness, craving, lacrimation, chills, vomiting. These effects are maximal 2–3 days after the abrupt withdrawal of heroin, morphine or related drugs.

102 (a) False (p. 428): cocaine is a major alkaloidal component from *Erythroxylon coca*. Leaves of this plant are chewed by Andean Indians to decrease the feeling of hunger and fatigue. Opium is from the dried juice from the seed capsule of the oriental poppy, *Papaver somniferum* (p. 420).
    (b) True (p. 428).
    (c) False (p. 428): 50 minutes. The half-life of amphetamine is 10 hours.
    (d) False (p. 428): 20%.
    (e) True (p. 429).

103 (a) False (pp. 435, 436): presynaptic agonist leading to decreased activity of 5-HT terminals in the forebrain.
    (b) True (p. 436): for example papillary dilatation, tachycardia, hyper-tension, hyper-reflexia, tremor, nausea, piloerection, hyperthermia.
    (c) True (p. 436): sensory modalities overlap.
    (d) True (p. 437): presumably because of desensitisation of the $5\text{-HT}_2$ receptors.
    (e) False (p. 437): no noticeable physical or psychological effects on abrupt withdrawal.

104 (a) True (p. 437): also hallucinogenic and analgesic properties.
    (b) True (p. 437): staggering gait, slurred speech, nystagmus.
    (c) True (pp. 437–438): also sweating and disorientation. Sometimes aggression.
    (d) True (p. 438): the individual may be unaware of violent acts on recovering from the effects of the drug.
    (e) True (p. 438).

105 With regard to cannabis and cannabinoids the following are true:
(a) The cannabinoid content of herbal cannabis is approximately 20%.
(b) Cannabis resin comprises up to 30% cannabinoids.
(c) The purest form of the drug produced for illicit use is cannabis oil.
(d) Tetrahydrocannabinol (THC) is believed to be the active ingredient.
(e) THC is metabolised to active metabolites in the liver.

106 Tolerance of and dependence on cannabinoids:
(a) Tolerance develops to the drug-induced mood changes.
(b) Tolerance develops to the effects of THC on psychomotor performance.
(c) Cross-tolerance occurs between cannabinoids and the psychotomimetics.
(d) Psychological dependence may arise.
(e) Physical dependence may arise.

107 Smoking a cigarette comprising 2% THC adversely affects:
(a) Memory.
(b) Motor coordination.
(c) Cognition.
(d) Sense of time.
(e) Mood.

108 Cannabinoids have the following pharmacological effects:
(a) Flashbacks.
(b) Hypotension.
(c) Bronchoconstriction.
(d) Lack of ovulation in females.
(e) Raised intraocular pressure.

109 The following drugs are paired correctly with the dermatological reaction:
(a) Tricyclic antidepressants and exanthematic reactions.
(b) Chlordiazepoxide and fixed eruption.
(c) Diazepam and photosensitivity reaction.
(d) Lithium and acneiform eruption.
(e) Imipramine and pigmentation.

105 (a) False (p. 440): up to approximately 8%. It varies according to the climate and growing conditions.
  (b) False (p. 440): up to 14%. Resin is an exudate secreted from the hairs on the leaves of the plants. The resinous material is powdered and usually compressed into a hard, brownish mass ('hash, 'resin', 'charas') which darkens in the air as a result of oxidation.
  (c) True (p. 440): up to 60% cannabinoids. This is prepared by solvent extraction of the resin followed by further purification.
  (d) True (p. 440).
  (e) True (p. 441): which are further metabolised to inactive polar compounds. These are excreted in the urine.

106 (a) True (p. 442): also to tachycardia, hyperthermia and decreased intraocular pressure.
  (b) True (p. 442): also to changes on EEG.
  (c) False (p. 442): alcohol and THC.
  (d) True (p. 442): as evidenced by withdrawal effects (irritability, insomnia, weight loss, tremor, changed sleep profile, anorexia) on abrupt withdrawal of the drug. Also holds for physical dependence.
  (e) True (p. 442).

  Note. Tissue tolerance, as opposed to metabolic tolerance, is the likely explanation for the effects noted.

107 (a) True (p. 442).
  (b) True (p. 442).
  (c) True (p. 442).
  (d) True (p. 442).
  (e) False (p. 442): euphoria.

108 (a) True (p. 442): have been reported in those exposed to high doses.
  (b) False (p. 443): hypertension, tachycardia.
  (c) False (p. 443): bronchodilatation.
  (d) True (p. 443): by suppressing release of luteinising hormone. There is some evidence that spermatogenesis and testosterone levels are decreased.
  (e) False (p. 443): lowers intraocular pressure, which may be beneficial in the treatment of glaucoma.

109 (a) False (p. 495): chlordiazepoxide and phenothiazines.
  (b) True (p. 495).
  (c) True (p. 495): also chlordiazepoxide, chlorpromazine, and protriptyline and other antidepressants.
  (d) True (p. 495): lithium is also associated with aggravation of psoriasis, and lupus-erythematosus-like syndrome.
  (e) False (p. 495): phenothiazines.

110 Ophthalmic effects of drugs:
(a) The antimuscarinic effect may cause cycloplegia.
(b) Phenothiazines cause pigmentation in the eye.
(c) Lenticular opacities occur with chlorpromazine.
(d) Glaucoma as a side-effect of psychotropics is not common.
(e) Pigmentary retinopathy occurs especially with thioridazines.

111 The following drug interactions and effects occur:
(a) Benzodiazepines interact with alpha-adrenergic blockers to cause an enhanced hypotensive effect.
(b) The metabolism of clonazepam is inhibited when combined with anti-epileptics.
(c) Diazepam metabolism is enhanced when combined with omeprazole.
(d) Benzodiazepine metabolism is inhibited when interacted with cimetidine.
(e) There is a transient enhancement of warfarin anticoagulant effect when combined with chloral.

112 The following MAOI interactions and effects are correct:
(a) Hypertensive crisis when combined with sympatomimetics.
(b) Decreased hypoglycaemic effect when combined with oral hypoglycaemics.
(c) Enhanced anticonvulsant effect of anti-epileptics.
(d) CNS toxicity in combination with SSRIs.
(e) CNS excitation with antipsychotics.

113 SSRI interactions:
(a) Enhanced anticoagulant effect of warfarin with all SSRIs.
(b) CNS toxicity with lithium.
(c) Increased plasma concentration of carbamazepine in combination with fluoxetine.
(d) Increased plasma concentration of propranolol in combination with fluvoxamine.
(e) Decreased plasma concentration of paroxetine in combination with phenytoin.

114 Tricyclic antidepressant interactions include:
(a) Antagonism of anticonvulsant effect of anti-epileptics.
(b) Increased hypotensive effect when combined with antihypertensives.
(c) Increased metabolism of tricyclics when combined with disulfiram.
(d) Decreased plasma concentration of theophylline when combined with tricyclic antidepressants.
(e) Increased plasma concentration of cimetidine when combined with tricyclic antidepressants.

110 (a)   True  (p. 496): also mydriasis.
  (b)   True  (p. 497): as well as in the skin. Pigmentation occurs in exposed parts of the bulbar conjunctiva and cornea, specks in the lens and pigmentary retinopathy.
  (c)   True  (p. 497).
  (d)   True  (p. 497).
  (e)   True  (p. 497): especially thioridazine in doses exceeding 800 mg/ day.

111 (a)   True  (p. 501).
  (b)   False (p. 501): accelerated metabolism.
  (c)   False (p. 501): inhibited metabolism.
  (d)   True  (p. 501).
  (e)   True  (p. 501).

112 (a)   True  (p. 502): also true when interacted with alcoholic and de-alcoholised beverages containing tyramine, and with L-dopa.
  (b)   False (p. 502): increased hypoglycaemic effect when combined with insulin, metformin and sulphonylureas.
  (c)   False (p. 502): antagonism of anticonvulsant effect.
  (d)   True  (p. 502).
  (e)   True  (p. 502): MAOIs also interact with antipsychotics to cause hypertension.

113 (a)   True  (p. 503).
  (b)   True  (p. 503).
  (c)   True  (p. 503).
  (d)   True  (p. 503).
  (e)   True  (p. 503).

114 (a)   True  (p. 504).
  (b)   True  (p. 504).
  (c)   False (p. 504): decreased metabolism.
  (d)   False (p. 504): increased.
  (e)   False (p. 504): increased plasma concentration of tricyclic anti-depressants.

115 The following antipsychotic interactions are correct:
(a) Increased absorption of phenothiazines with antacids.
(b) Increased metabolism of haloperidol with rifampicin.
(c) Accelerated metabolism of clozapine in combination with phenytoin.
(d) Increased risk of extrapyramidal effects in combination with metoclopramide.
(e) Decreased plasma concentration of chlorpromazine in combination with propranolol.

116 Lithium interactions include:
(a) Increased risk of lithium toxicity with metronidazole.
(b) Increased theophylline excretion.
(c) Neurotoxicity with verapamil.
(d) Occasional impairment of glucose tolerance with antidiabetic drugs.
(e) Antagonism of cholinergic effect with cholinergics.

115 (a)  False (p. 505): decreased absorption.
    (b)  True (p. 505).
    (c)  True (p. 505).
    (d)  True (p. 505).
    (e)  False (p. 505): increased plasma chlorpromazine.

116 (a)  True (p. 506).
    (b)  False (p. 506): increased lithium excretion, when lithium interacts
         with theophylline
    (c)  True (p. 506).
    (d)  True (p. 506).
    (e)  True (p. 506).

# Practical Forensic Psychiatry

1   The following are true statements:
(a)  Males between 10 and 20 years of age account for approximately half of all recorded crime.
(b)  Many juvenile offenders have an ICD–10 diagnosis.
(c)  The age of criminal responsibility is 8 years in Scotland.
(d)  The most common type of offence is acquisitive offence.
(e)  Violent crime accounts for only 5% of the total.

2   The following statements are true:
(a)  The male:female ratio for recorded crime is 10:1.
(b)  Women are more likely to commit offences of theft and fraud.
(c)  The age distribution of female offenders is similar to that of males.
(d)  Cautioning is the main disposal used for female offenders.
(e)  In the UK matricide appears to be more common than patricide.

3   For the legal definition of murder to be fulfilled the following criteria must met:
(a)  The offender must be over 10 years of age.
(b)  The offender is not suffering from mental illness.
(c)  The offender had intent.
(d)  There is an absence of immediate severe provocation.
(e)  There is proof of unlawful or negligent behaviour.

4   With reference to homicide the following are true:
(a)  The victim is known to the offender in approximately half of homicides.
(b)  In 25% of cases the victim is related to the offender or is a lover.
(c)  Approximately 40% of all victims of homicide are children.
(d)  When children are victims, those under 1 year are most at risk.
(e)  The killing of a parent is the rarest of intrafamilial homicide.

5   The following are true statements:
(a)  Psychiatric factors are more often described in female than male homicides.
(b)  Women are responsible for over one-third of all homicides in which the offender has a psychiatric disorder.
(c)  Women predominate among depressive homicides.
(d)  In men the conjunction of psychosis and homicide tends to occur in the older age group.
(e)  Sadistic aggressive acts are more likely to occur in response to a need to bolster low self-esteem.

1   (a) True (p. 14): the peak age for offending is in the age group 14–17 years.
    (b) False (p. 14): few have attracted a psychiatric diagnosis.
    (c) True (p. 14): but in England and Wales it is 10 years.
    (d) True (p. 15): that is, property offences.
    (e) True (p. 15): including violence against the person, sexual offences and robbery.

2   (a) False (p. 17): the ratio is 5:1 – 17% of known offenders are female, but the male:female ratio varies for different types of crime.
    (b) True (p. 17): some crimes, for example soliciting for prostitution, are commited mainly by women; other offences, especially sexual crimes, but also burglary and violent crimes, are commited predominantly by men.
    (c) True (p. 17): the age distribution of female offenders is similar to that of males, partly, but with a secondary peak of middle-aged shoplifters.
    (d) True (p. 17): half of female offenders, a third of males.
    (e) True (p. 20): this differs in other countries.

3   (a) True (p. 18): homicide is said to be murder when the offender is of sound mind and discretion (over the age of 10), and had malice aforethought (i.e. the intent to cause death or grievous bodily harm).
    (b) True (p. 18): "Is of sound mind and discretion and had malice aforethought".
    (c) True (p. 18).
    (d) True (p. 19): this is a mitigating factor for manslaughter.
    (e) False (p. 19): Such behaviour gives grounds for manslaughter.

4   (a) False (p. 20): approximately 75% in British studies.
    (b) False (p. 20): approximately 50%.
    (c) False (p. 20): approximately 15%, the commonest victims being children under 1 year. Males are generally at more risk than females.
    (d) True (p. 20).
    (e) True (p. 20): the killing of a parent accounts for less than 5% of all homicides.

5   (a) True (pp.20–21): in approximately 70% of female homicides the offender had a psychiatric disorder compared with 30% of male homicides.
    (b) True (p. 21): but women are responsible for only 2% of 'normal' homicides in which the conviction was for murder.
    (c) True (p. 21): the commonest victim is their child.
    (d) False (p. 21): it is the conjunction of depression and homicide.
    (e) True (p. 22).

6  A typical profile of an offender of multiple victims is as follows:
(a)  Suffering from a psychotic illness.
(b)  Black ethnic origin.
(c)  Age 40–50 years.
(d)  Socio-economic group 1–2.
(e)  Tends to pick strangers as victims.


7  With reference to the killing of infants and children the following are true statements:
(a)  Sexual offenders comprise approximately 40% of the total group of homicide offenders.
(b)  Of child victims under 1 year, 90% are killed by their mother.
(c)  Infanticide is the killing of a child under 12 months by a parent.
(d)  Neonaticide is the killing of a baby less than 6 weeks old.
(e)  The 'Medea complex' refers to the infanticide in which there is a desire to punish the spouse by killing the children.


8  Factitious illness by proxy has the following features:
(a)  The perpetrator is equally likely to be the father or mother.
(b)  The perpetrator frequently has nursing experience.
(c)  In approximately 50% of cases there is a history of factitious illness behaviour in the mother.
(d)  Commonly the father is emotionally if not physically absent.
(e)  The perpetrator often appears to be an exemplary mother.


9  Child-stealing by women:
(a)  'Comforting offences' are carried out by older women generally who suffer from personality disorders.
(b)  'Manipulative offences' are carried out by older women with personality disorder.
(c)  'Impulsive psychotic offences' are usually carried out during the acute relapse of a psychotic illness.
(d)  There is a small risk of repetition.
(e)  Most abducted babies are found quickly, well cared for and unharmed.


10  Child sexual abuse:
(a)  It is estimated that 10–15% of female children have been victims of unequivocal sexual assault.
(b)  Sexual intercourse under 16 years is regarded in law as statutory rape.
(c)  Paedophiles who lack acceptance of the deleterious effects of their sexual behaviour with children are very resistant to change.
(d)  Abusers typically display distorted perceptions and attitudes.
(e)  Family relationships which do not involve consanguinity generally do not fall within the legal definition of incest.

6   (a) False (p. 22): there is a paucity of literature on this, partly because of the rarity of such cases and because the offenders frequently commit suicide after the killing. However, a typical profile is of a non-psychotic White male, around 20–30 years of age, of socio-economic group 3–4, who uses a firearm in a dramatic scenario to express resentment and anger at life's frustrations and his personal difficulties. Some serial killers are psychotically motivated, though.
    (b) False (p. 22): they are White. The ratio of 10:1 Black to White applies to perpetrators with *single* victims (p. 23).
    (c) False (p. 22): aged 20–30 years.
    (d) False (p. 22): socio-economic group 3–4.
    (e) True (p. 23).

7   (a) False (p. 23): sexual offenders comprise about 20% of the total group of homicide offenders; 80% are parents or parent substitutes.
    (b) False (p. 23): approximately 60% are killed by their mother.
    (c) False (p. 23): infanticide is the killing of a child under 12 months by a mother.
    (d) False (p. 23): neonaticide is the killing of a baby less than 1 day old.
    (e) True (p. 24).

8   (a) False (p. 26): mother.
    (b) True (p. 26).
    (c) False (p. 26): approximately one-third.
    (d) True (p. 26): and oblivious to what is going on.
    (e) True (p. 26).

9   (a) False (p. 27): the profile is of a young woman, motivated by a desire to satisfy her need to look after a young child. She is more likely to take a child she has already known (e.g. through babysitting) and have a history of her own children being taken into care. Frequently she will have a history of delinquency and emotional deprivation and a diagnosis of personality disorder.
    (b) True (p. 27): the baby is stolen for a particular purpose, for example to maintain a relationship by claiming the baby was her partner's or to replace one lost by miscarriage.
    (c) True (p. 27).
    (d) True (p. 27): especially in emotionally deprived women with a hysterical personality who are preoccupied with their desire to have children.
    (e) True (p. 27).

10  (a) True (p. 30): 5–8% will have experienced sexual intercourse.
    (b) False (p. 30): under 13 years.
    (c) True (p. 32): also, unless methods of self-control are developed, reoffending is common.
    (d) True (p. 32).
    (e) True (p. 32).

11   Incest:
(a)   Consent is occasionally a statutory defence to the charge.
(b)   The legal definition requires that sexual intercourse occurs.
(c)   Father–daughter incest usually takes place when the girl is aged about 4 or 5 years.
(d)   The father who has an incestuous relationship with his daughter usually suffers from a psychiatric abnormality.
(e)   Mother–son incest is often associated with neurotic states and personality difficulties.

12   Possible side-effects of cyproterone acetate include:
(a)   Asthenia.
(b)   Lassitude.
(c)   Gynaecomastia.
(d)   Inhibition of spermatogenesis and erection.
(e)   Elation.

13   Violent sexual offences:
(a)   Approximately 90% of rapists do not commit a second rape.
(b)   The majority of rapists fail to ejaculate during the act.
(c)   Many rapists suffer relative impotence during the act.
(d)   It is believed that the great majority of perpetrators of sexual crimes begin their offending behaviour in adolescence.
(e)   Some 20% of victims develop chronic anxiety and depressive symptoms.

14   Exhibitionism:
(a)   Is a paraphilia.
(b)   80% of first offenders reoffend.
(c)   Characteristically takes place at a distance.
(d)   Rooth described an inhibited but apparently normal personality type.
(e)   The offenders often suffer from learning difficulties.

15   Shoplifters:
(a)   Recent studies suggest that it affects the genders equally.
(b)   Psychiatric disorder is a factor in a small number.
(c)   One peak age is 70–80 years.
(d)   It is a recognised occurrence in organic states such as epilepsy.
(e)   Depressive pseudo-dementia may be a defence.

11   (a)   False (p.32): consent is not a defence to the charge.
     (b)   True (p. 32): incest is when a man has sexual intercourse with a female whom he knows to be his daughter, granddaughter, sister, half-sister or mother, or when a woman aged over 16 years permits a man whom she knows to be of such consanguity to have sexual intercourse with her. Family relationships which do not involve consanguity, for example stepfather–daughter, do not fall within the legal definition in England and Wales.
     (c)   False (p. 32): 10 or 11 or earlier.
     (d)   False (p. 33): rarely suffers from a psychiatric disorder, although he frequently shows evidence of personality difficulties and inadequacies.
     (e)   True (p. 33): or occasionally psychosis.

12   (a)   True (p. 37).
     (b)   True (p. 37).
     (c)   True (p. 37).
     (d)   True (p. 37).
     (e)   False (p. 37): depression.

     Note. Antilibinal medication requires the patient's compliance and consent. Additional side-effects include weight changes.

13   (a)   True (p. 38): although 15% in one study were convicted of a further sexual assault and 17% of a violent offence. Reoffending correlated positively with the number of previous offences and inversely with the age of the offender. However, sexual offenders against children are more likely to reoffend.
     (b)   True (p. 34): nor is emission necessary for the legal definition of rape.
     (c)   True (p. 34).
     (d)   True (pp. 36–37): Frequently in their early teens or even earlier.
     (e)   True (p. 38): which may occur after a delay of many years. Victims of rape are susceptible to short- and long-term traumatic after-effects.

14   (a)   True (p. 39).
     (b)   False (p. 39): do not reoffend.
     (c)   True (p. 40): and no physical contact takes place.
     (d)   True (p. 40): but also an overtly aggressive and antisocial type.
     (e)   False (p. 39): rarely suffer from learning disability, schizophrenia, mania or an organic disorder.

15   (a)   True (p. 41): or greater numbers of men.
     (b)   True (p. 42): approximately 5% suffer from substantial mental disorder.
     (c)   False (p. 42): peaks in 50–60-year age group and teenagers.
     (d)   True (p. 42): either in the confusional period following an epileptic attack or in association with an abnormal personality.
     (e)   True (p. 42).

16 The following are recognised fire-setting subgroups:
(a) A sizeable proportion are sexually aroused by the act.
(b) Those motivated by revenge, self-protection or anger.
(c) Psychotic illness accounts for a significant proportion of offenders.
(d) Those seeking the release of tension.
(e) Gang members as part of gang activity (with a low rate of recidivism).

17 The following statements are true of the relationship between crime and schizophrenia:
(a) People with schizophrenia show a similar rate of offending to the rest of the population.
(b) People with schizophrenia are more likely to commit a crime of violence than the rest of the population.
(c) People with schizophrenia are more likely than other offenders to be arrested.
(d) For first admission with schizophrenia, violence preceding admission is uncommon.
(e) Patients with schizophrenia with negative symptoms generally commit occasional but often well-planned and serious violence.

18 The following are true statements with regard to offending behaviour:
(a) Assaults by people with schizophrenia are mostly against victims they already know.
(b) Delusional ideas often motivate an act.
(c) Command hallucinations are frequently disclosed in mental state examination before the act.
(d) The most commonly assaulted stranger is the arresting police officer after a public order offence.
(e) Usually the persistence of normal aspects of personality acts as a break on aggressive behaviour.

19 Affective disorders and offending:
(a) Offending is less common than in other functional psychosis.
(b) A stranger is the usual victim in altruistic homicides.
(c) Offending is more common in mania and hypomania than in depression.
(d) Violent offending in depressive disorders is rare but may be serious.
(e) People with manic–depressive disorder are more likely to be violent to themselves than others.

20 Of serious sexual offences the following are true:
(a) The motivation is often principally for sexual gratification.
(b) The psychopathology is usually that of unresolved aggressive feelings about significant female figures.
(c) There is often a history of cold and affectionless upbringing by unloving parents.
(d) There is often a history of a violent father and an over-involved mother.
(e) There is often a history of persistent uncertainties about sexual orientation.

16  (a)  False (p. 45): a very small proportion of the total.
    (b)  True  (p. 45): makes up at least half of the total referred for psychiatric assessment.
    (c)  False (p. 46): small minority.
    (d)  True  (p. 45): the principal motivation for the fire-setter is the relief of despondency and tension by the act of setting a fire.
    (e)  True  (p. 45): low rate of recidivism except for the leader.

        Note. Fire-setting by women is less common.


17  (a)  True  (p. 53).
    (b)  True  (pp. 53–54): usually minor in degree.
    (c)  True  (p. 54): also to be detected.
    (d)  False (p. 54): it is common in this group.
    (e)  False (p. 54): offences committed inadvertently or neglectfully.

        Note. People with schizophrenia are over-represented among violent offenders and violent inpatients (p. 58).


18  (a)  True  (p. 57): assaultive crimes by people with schizophrenia are mostly against victims they already know.
    (b)  True  (p. 56): half the sample of one study had acted on their delusions, although violent acts were uncommon.
    (c)  False (p. 56): command hallucinations are frequently disclosed in mental state examination after the act.
    (d)  True  (p. 57).
    (e)  True  (p. 55): especially in those not habitually prone to using violence to resolve interpersonal difficulties.


19  (a)  True  (p. 64).
    (b)  False (p. 64): family member.
    (c)  True  (p. 64): and may be serious.
    (d)  True  (p. 64).
    (e)  True  (p. 61).


20  (a)  False (p. 69): the offence is often about revenge, destruction or release of tension.
    (b)  True  (p. 69): often the mother, for whom the victim becomes a surrogate or even a representation of all women.
    (c)  True  (p. 69).
    (d)  True  (p. 69).
    (e)  True  (p. 69): also a history of institutional rearing, sexual abuse, all in a setting of marked psychological disturbance and low self-esteem.

21   The following are true statements:

(a)   Antisocial behaviour often appears before any sign of neurological or psychiatric disturbances in Huntington's chorea.
(b)   The prevalence of epilepsy among prisoners is twice that in the general population.
(c)   There is an excess of violent crimes in epileptic prisoners.
(d)   Violence resulting directly from epileptic activity is rare.
(e)   Violence in epilepsy is usually a non-goal-directed activity in the ictal phase.

22   The following are true statements:

(a)   Psychotic morbid jealousy shows a poorer response to treatment than neurotic morbid jealousy.
(b)   De Clerambault's syndrome is often monodelusional.
(c)   To fund their peregrinations people with Munchhausen's syndrome may commit thefts and create disturbances.
(d)   Pathological gambling is more generally associated with recidivism and other delinquent activity.
(e)   Gambling is highest in young offenders.

23   The following abilities are the essential criteria with regard to fitness to plead:

(a)   Instruct a lawyer.
(b)   Object to selection of a juror.
(c)   Plead to the charge.
(d)   Understand the charge.
(e)   Understand the evidence.

24   The following are true statements:

(a)   Most criminal acts require evidence of *mens rea*.
(b)   The absence of *mens rea* forms the basis of the defence of automatism.
(c)   Legal automatism has no relationship to the clinical concept of automatic behaviour.
(d)   If the offending behaviour can recur it is labelled insane automatism.
(e)   Insane automatism requires behaviours caused by brain diseases (e.g. tumours and epilepsy).

25   Automatisms:

(a)   Sane automatisms are once-only events.
(b)   Sane automatisms are said to be due to internal causes.
(c)   Sane automatisms include night terrors.
(d)   Sane automatisms may include sleepwalking.
(e)   May include the post-ictal confusional states.

21 (a) True (p. 76).
   (b) True (p. 76): but not greatly different from the rate found in most disadvantaged socio-economic groups.
   (c) False (p. 76): there is no excess – the rate and type of offending in epileptics are similar to those of offenders in general.
   (d) True (p. 76).
   (e) False (p. 76): violence in epilepsy is usually non-goal-directed activity in the post-ictal phase. Ictal violence is uncommon.

22 (a) False (p. 79): better than neurotic morbid jealousy.
   (b) False (p. 80): usually associated with a paranoid psychosis or schizophrenia.
   (c) True (p. 80).
   (d) True (p. 81).
   (e) True (p. 81).

23 (a) True (p. 108).
   (b) True (p. 108): more usually accepted as 'challenge' a juror.
   (c) True (p. 108): understand the difference between saying guilty and not guilty.
   (d) True (p. 108).
   (e) True (p. 108).

   Note. The issue of fitness to plead is normally determined by a jury (p. 114). The jury bases its decision on the written or oral evidence of two or more medical practitioners, at least one of whom is approved under section 12 of the Mental Health Act 1983.

24 (a) True (p. 120): almost every criminal offence requires *mens rea* (or 'guilty mind'). If the mind does not have the potential to control physical acts, there is an absence of *mens rea* and this forms the basis of the defence of automatism (see question 25).
   (b) True (p. 120).
   (c) True (p. 120).
   (d) True (p. 120).
   (e) True (p. 121).

25 (a) True (p. 121).
   (b) False (p. 121): there are external causes.
   (c) True (p. 121): also confusional states and concussion, and reflex actions following, for example, bee stings, dissociative states, hypoglycaemia.
   (d) False (p. 121): this is an insane automatism.
   (e) False (p. 121): these are insane automatisms.

26   With reference to dangerousness:

(a)   Previous similar behaviour has primacy as a statistical predictor of future violence.
(b)   An older offender is more likely to commit future acts of violence.
(c)   Property offenders are most likely to reoffend.
(d)   Shorter length of stay in special hospital has been shown to be associated with a lesser likelihood of reoffending.
(e)   Less reoffending occurs with conditional than with absolute discharge.


27   The Care Programme Approach requires:

(a)   A discharge plan.
(b)   Monthly review.
(c)   Consultation with users.
(d)   A nominated key social worker.
(e)   Systematic assessment of health and social care needs.


28   Psychiatry in prison:

(a)   Women have fewer previous convictions than men.
(b)   Women are more likely to have committed a drug offence than men.
(c)   Over 50% of female prisoners have a psychiatric disorder.
(d)   Behavioural disorder is more common in females than males.
(e)   Females are put 'on report' for offences in prison at twice the rate of men.


29   Suicide in prisons:

(a)   The annual rate has been consistent over the past 100 years.
(b)   It is the second commonest mode of death in prisons.
(c)   The rate is close to 10 times that found in the general population.
(d)   Suicide is most common in 'life' prisoners.
(e)   Suicide is nearly always achieved by drug overdose.

26  (a) True (pp. 216, 217): type and quantity of previous offending are the most powerful predictors of future offending.
    (b) False (pp. 216, 217): younger age is the second strongest correlate for reoffending.
    (c) True (p. 217).
    (d) False (p. 217): it is associated with a greater likelihood of reoffending, but this may be confounded by the influence of age.
    (e) True (p. 217).

> Note. Diagnosis, severity of disorder and personality traits are the poorest predictors of violence (p. 219). Violent offenders are more likely to reoffend with violence, and homicidal offenders are less likely to reoffend than other violent offenders (p. 217). More offending occurs in psychopathic disorder than in other mental illnesses. Alcohol and drug misuse probably increases the likelihood of reoffending. Unemployment, an unstable family background and poor education/low intelligence are generally associated with reoffending.

27  (a) False (p. 226): not specific enough – requires a written care plan.
    (b) False (p. 226): regular review, time interval not specified.
    (c) True (p. 226).
    (d) False (p. 226): a key worker.
    (e) True (p. 226).

28  (a) True (p. 255).
    (b) True (p. 255): also less likely to have committed a crime of violence or burglary, and are more likely to have committed a drug offence, theft, fraud or deception. In the past decade there has been a sharp rise in the number of women serving sentences for drug trafficking.
    (c) True (p. 255).
    (d) True (p. 255): particularly among those on remand or serving a short sentence.
    (e) True (p. 255).

29  (a) False (p. 259): in fact, it doubled within the 1990s.
    (b) False (p. 259): it is the commonest.
    (c) True (p. 259).
    (d) False (p. 259): in remand prisoners.
    (e) False (p. 259): hanging.

# Psychosexual Disorders

1    The following are matched correctly:
(a)    Ventral striatal dopamine-dependent mechanisms and sexual appetite behaviour.
(b)    Amygdala and sexual appetite behaviour.
(c)    Steroidal hormones and sexual appetite behaviour and copulation.
(d)    Copulation and the medial pre-optic area.
(e)    Copulation and the hypothalamus.

2    The following are true of oxytocin:
(a)    The neurohypophysis secretes a pulse of oxytocin at orgasm.
(b)    Oxytocin is implicated in social bonding.
(c)    Oxytocin can induce sexual arousal in females.
(d)    Paraventricular nucleus neurons containing oxytocin project to the autonomic centres in the spinal cord, regulating blood flow to the genitals.
(e)    Oxytocin can be given intranasally to facilitate breast-feeding.

3    The following are true of the spinal mechanisms and pathways in sexual function:
(a)    Vasocongestion is a result of increased sympathetic outflow.
(b)    Erections can occur in men with complete spinal cord lesions above the sacral segments.
(c)    Bilateral cordotomy at the upper thoracic levels sometimes results in loss of erectile ability.
(d)    The brain-stem principally has an inhibitory influence on spinal mechanisms regulating erection.
(e)    Parasympathetic outflow is responsible for increased vaginal transudate.

4    The following peripheral mechanisms are important in genital arousal:
(a)    Parasympathetic activity causes dilatation of the arterioles supplying erectile tissue.
(b)    Parasympathetic activity causes contraction of trabecular smooth muscle.
(c)    Venous occlusion is probably by mechanical means and not neurally mediated.
(d)    Acetylcholine is involved in mediating sympathetic effects on penile tumescence.
(e)    Vasoactive intestinal polypeptide plays a major role in erection.

1   (a) True (p. 2).
    (b) True (p. 2).
    (c) True (p. 2).
    (d) True (p. 2).
    (e) True (p. 2).

2   (a) True (p. 4).
    (b) True (p. 4).
    (c) True (p. 4).
    (d) True (p. 4).
    (e) True (p. 4).

3   (a) False (p. 5): parasympathetic.
    (b) True (p. 5): entirely reflex erection.
    (c) False (p. 5): most men.
    (d) False (p. 5): excitatory and inhibitory.
    (e) True (p. 5).

4   (a) True (p. 6).
    (b) False (p. 6): relaxation.
    (c) True (p. 7): although some believe there is some neural input.
    (d) False (p. 7): parasympathetic.
    (e) True (p. 7).

5    The following are true of the peripheral mechanisms in sexual activity:

(a)  Sympathetic outflow from T6 to L6 segments of the spinal cord tonically inhibit erection.
(b)  Sympathetic outflow tonically inhibits erection and causes vasocongestion.
(c)  Alpha antagonists when injected intracavernosally induce a flaccid state.
(d)  The flaccid state is maintained through the activation of presynaptic alpha$_1$ adrenoceptors.
(e)  Increased sympathetic tone is believed to be implicated in anxiety-induced impotence.

6    The following are true of the somatomotor mechanism of sexual activity:

(a)  Penile sensory fibres belong to the spinal segments S2 to S5.
(b)  Penile sensory fibres travel in a branch of the perineal nerve.
(c)  The dorsal nerve of the penis and penile sensory fibres form the afferent pathways for reflex erection.
(d)  The nucleus of Onufrowicz is part of the somatomotor mechanism.
(e)  The bulbocavernous reflex results in intracavernosal pressure above systolic blood pressure.

7    The following are correctly paired:

(a)  Acetylcholine and vasoconstriction.
(b)  Relaxing factor and nitric oxide.
(c)  Prostaglandins and cavernosal muscle relaxation.
(d)  Prostacyclin and vasodilatation.
(e)  Vasoactive intestinal peptide and vasoconstriction.

8    The following statements are correct:

(a)  There is no correlation between circulating testosterone levels and measures of sexual interest in men.
(b)  Testosterone can increase sexual appetite in women.
(c)  Oophorectomy reduces oestrogen and androgen production by 50%.
(d)  Oestrogens are more important than androgens in determining a woman's sexual appetite.
(e)  The main metabolites of testosterone are oestradiol and dihydrotestosterone.

9    The following are correctly linked with an erection:

(a)  Apomorphine induces erections.
(b)  D$_1$ receptor agonists and induction of erections.
(c)  Aspermia and alpha adrenoceptor antagonists.
(d)  Drugs that increase central serotonergic neurotransmission and a reduction in sexual activity.
(e)  Drugs causing priapism and peripheral alpha adrenoceptor agonists.

5   (a) False (p. 8): T11 to L3.
    (b) False (p. 8): causes detumescence.
    (c) False (p. 8): penile tumescence.
    (d) False (p. 8): postsynaptic.
    (e) True (p. 8).

6   (a) False (p. 8): spinal segments S2 to S4.
    (b) False (p. 8): dorsal nerve of the penis, a branch of the pudendal
        nerve.
    (c) True (p. 8).
    (d) True (p. 8): motor neurons supply the ischiocavernosus and
        bulbocavernosus and form a group of the grey column of the spinal
        cord.
    (e) True (p. 9).

7   (a) False (p. 9): vasodilatation.
    (b) True (p. 9).
    (c) True (p. 10).
    (d) True (p. 10).
    (e) False (p. 7): erection.

8   (a) True (p. 10): nor activity, nor erectile function.
    (b) True (p. 10).
    (c) True (p. 11).
    (d) False (p. 11): the reverse is true.
    (e) True (p. 12).

9   (a) True (p. 13): apamorphine does induce erections.
    (b) False (p. 13): $D_2$ receptor agonists and induction of erections.
    (c) True (p. 14): aspermia or failure to ejaculate at orgasm is linked with
        side-effects of alpha adrenoceptor antagonists, and occurs in one-
        third of men taking thioridazine.
    (d) True (p. 14).
    (e) False (p. 15): blockade.

10 Decreased sexual appetite is a well-recognised finding in the following conditions:
(a) Hypothalamo-pituitary disease.
(b) Multiple sclerosis.
(c) Temporal lobe epilepsy.
(d) Spinal cord lesions.
(e) Hypoprolactinaemia.

11 The following are correct:
(a) Prenatal androgenisation is likely to affect the formation of gender identity.
(b) Individuals with complete androgen insensitivity syndrome will still develop a male gender identity.
(c) Gender identity is probably determined by psychological rather than biological factors.
(d) Prenatal androgens predispose towards masculine gender role behaviour.
(e) Progesterones are more likely to have a feminising influence on gender-role behaviour.

12 The following are true statements:
(a) The traditional psychoanalytical theory states that gender development is rooted in the phallic stage of psychosexual development at 3 years of age.
(b) Gender-typed behaviour is thought to result from the differential reinforcement of boys and girls.
(c) Social learning theorists state that boys and girls learn gender-typed behaviour by imitating models of the same gender.
(d) According to cognitive development theorists a basic gender identity is established by 9 years of age.
(e) Gender schemas influence the way in which we perceive and remember information.

13 The age at which puberty begins is influenced by the following factors:
(a) Geographical location.
(b) Ethnicity.
(c) Genetic factors.
(d) Emotional state.
(e) Birth order.

14 The following are true of the time sequence of puberty:
(a) An upsurge in the production of follicle-stimulating hormone (FSH) is the first hormonal change.
(b) The growth of pubic hair is the first physical sign.
(c) Menstruation occurs when a critical percentage of body fat has been reached.
(d) In boys puberty begins 3 years later on average than in girls.
(e) A rapid growth spurt in boys heralds puberty.

10   (a)  True  (p. 22).
     (b)  True  (p. 22).
     (c)  True  (p. 21).
     (d)  False (pp. 22, 23): erectile dysfunction.
     (e)  False (p. 26): hyperprolactinaemia.

11   (a)  False (p. 31).
     (b)  False (p. 32): female gender identity in spite of the Y chromosome.
     (c)  True  (p. 32).
     (d)  True  (pp. 32–33).
     (e)  False (p. 33): can be either masculinising or feminising.

12   (a)  False (p. 34): this occurs at 5 years.
     (b)  True  (p. 36).
     (c)  True  (p. 37).
     (d)  False (p. 38): it occurs at 2–3 years.
     (e)  True  (p. 39).

13   (a)  True  (p. 39).
     (b)  True  (p. 39).
     (c)  True  (p. 39).
     (d)  True  (p. 39).
     (e)  False (p. 39).

14   (a)  False (p. 39): gonadotrophin-releasing hormone.
     (b)  False (p. 39): body fat, breasts develop.
     (c)  True  (p. 39).
     (d)  False (p. 39): 2 years.
     (e)  False (p. 39): other physical changes predate this.

15  Compounds used in intracavernosal injections include:

(a)  Phentolamine.
(b)  Papaverine.
(c)  Prostaglandin E.
(d)  Vasoactive intestinal peptide.
(e)  Yohimbine.

16  Premature ejaculation:

(a)  Affects 15% of men.
(b)  Is best addressed by the 'stop–start' technique, as per Masters and Johnson.
(c)  Clomipramine delays ejaculation.
(d)  Selective serotonin reuptake inhibitors (SSRIs) cause premature ejaculation as a side-effect.
(e)  Is less likely than erectile dysfunction to be represented as a problem in sexual dysfunction clinics.

17  Delayed ejaculation:

(a)  Delayed ejaculation often presents as infertility.
(b)  It is easier to treat than premature ejaculation.
(c)  Masters and Johnson prescribed super-stimulation as treatment.
(d)  Yohimbine may assist ejaculation.
(e)  Delayed ejaculation is as common a complaint as premature ejaculation.

18  Male erectile disorders:

(a)  Erectile disorder is the commonest sexual dysfunction in men.
(b)  Transdermal nitrate patches to the penis may result in partner headaches.
(c)  Yohimbine works by increasing sympathetic and parasympathetic activity.
(d)  Testosterone is helpful in patients with hypogonadal states.
(e)  Alprostadil's mode of action is by smooth muscle relaxation.

19  The following statements are true of testosterone in relation to the treatment of male erectile dysfunction:

(a)  Erections in response to an external erotic stimulus will improve.
(b)  Benign prostatic hypertrophy must be excluded before prescription.
(c)  Treatments can be administered orally, intramuscularly or transdermally.
(d)  Patients must be warned of the risk of baldness.
(e)  Osteoporosis prevention should be considered in the risk–benefit analysis.

20  The most common side-effects of yohimbine are:

(a)  Anxiety.
(b)  Agitation.
(c)  Priapism.
(d)  Diarrhoea.
(e)  Influenza-like symptoms.

15  (a)  True (p. 78).
    (b)  True (p. 78).
    (c)  True (p. 78).
    (d)  True (p. 78).
    (e)  False (p. 78): it is an orally administered compound.

16  (a)  False (p. 79): 25%.
    (b)  False (p. 79): the 'squeeze' technique, as per Semans, and Masters
         and Johnson.
    (c)  True (p. 80).
    (d)  False (p. 80): delay ejaculation.
    (e)  True (p. 79).

17  (a)  True (p. 80).
    (b)  False (p. 80): more difficult.
    (c)  True (p. 80): also desipramine and eostigamine (p. 89).
    (d)  True (p. 80).
    (e)  False (p. 80): much rarer.

18  (a)  False (p. 84): but it is the most likely to present to clinical practice.
    (b)  True (pp.84–85): via transvaginal absorption. Also headaches in
         males.
    (c)  False (p. 85): presynaptic alpha$_2$ adrenergic receptor blocker
         increases parasympathetic (cholinergic) and decreases sympathetic
         (adrenergic) activity. 40% success rate.
    (d)  True (p. 85).
    (e)  True (p. 86): intracavernosal injection.

19  (a)  False (p. 86): not affected.
    (b)  False (p. 86): prostatic cancer.
    (c)  True (p. 86): or implants.
    (d)  True (p. 86): also decreased spermatogenesis.
    (e)  True (p. 86).

20  (a)  True (p. 85).
    (b)  True (p. 85).
    (c)  False (p. 85).
    (d)  True (p. 85).
    (e)  True (p. 85).

21 The side-effects of the intracavernosal injection of alprostadil include:
(a) Local haematomas.
(b) Transient hypotension.
(c) Local fibrosis.
(d) Tolerance.
(e) Visual disturbances.

22 Measures to effect detumescence in the event of prolonged erection include:
(a) Running up and down the stairs.
(b) Aspiration of 100–200 ml of blood from the corpora cavernosum.
(c) Topical application of ice packs.
(d) Local injection of vasoconstrictive agents such as phenylephedrine.
(e) Lowering of blood pressure by systemic agents.

23 The following are true with regard to drugs which are known to impair erections:
(a) The antidepressants desipramine and fluvoxamine are least likely to cause sexual dysfunction.
(b) As many as 60% of patients receiving thioridazine report sexual dysfunction.
(c) Benzodiazepines are believed to have little effect on sexual function.
(d) Beta blockers cause a reduction in serum testosterone.
(e) Lithium has been reported to cause male erectile dysfunction and a decrease in libido.

24 The following are true in relation to child abuse:
(a) There is a strong relationship between abuse and low socio-economic status.
(b) Characteristics of the child such as chronic physical illness may increase the risk.
(c) Child abuse has been linked with disorders of attention span.
(d) Intelligence is believed to be a protective factor against abuse.
(e) Intergenerational transmission of abuse is likely.

25 The non-organic psychiatric manifestations of infection with HIV include:
(a) Minor morbidity in a majority.
(b) Psychotic illnesses.
(c) Eating disorders.
(d) Sexual dysfunction.
(e) Major affective disorder in a sizeable proportion.

21  (a) True (p. 87).
    (b) True (p. 87): light-headedness and dizziness.
    (c) True (p. 87).
    (d) False (p. 87): not reported.˙
    (e) False (p. 87): noted with Viagra.

22  (a) True (p. 87): to encourage arterial shunting.
    (b) False (p. 88): 60 ml.
    (c) True (p. 87).
    (d) True (p. 88).
    (e) False (p. 88): not recognised.

23  (a) True (p. 93): also bupropion.
    (b) True (p. 93).
    (c) True (p. 93).
    (d) True (p. 93).
    (e) True (p. 93).

24  (a) True (p. 103).
    (b) True (p. 103).
    (c) True (p. 105): also language disorders.
    (d) True (p. 105).
    (e) False (p. 105): although this is a much-debated concept.

25  (a) True (p. 114): adjustment disorders, anxiety, transitory depression.
    (b) True (p. 115).
    (c) True (p. 115).
    (d) True (p. 115).
    (e) False (p. 115): a minority.

26 HIV and brain diseases:

(a) HIV enters the central nervous system (CNS) late in the infection.
(b) In the absence of significant neurological syndrome neuropathological abnormalities are unlikely.
(c) Neurological and neuropsychiatric symptoms develop in more than 80% of cases of advanced HIV disease.
(d) Mostly the CNS manifestations of HIV are secondary to the immune deficiency.
(e) At least 30% of people with AIDS develop dementia.

27 The following are correct of the neuropathology of HIV disease:

(a) HIV enters the brain within the first few months of infection.
(b) Up to 90% of people who die of AIDS show neuropathological abnormalities.
(c) There is macroscopic evidence of cerebral oedema.
(d) There is no correlation between the neuropathological changes and the severity of the clinical picture.
(e) HIV causes a distinct encephalitis.

28 The neuroradiology of HIV brain disease is as follows:

(a) Widening of the cortical sulci is detected.
(b) Computed tomography (CT) shows white matter pallor.
(c) Neuroradiology findings correlate well with the severity of the clinical picture.
(d) Neuroradiology proves useful in the differential diagnosis of opportunistic infections.
(e) Positron emission tomography (PET) and single-photon emission computed tomography (SPECT) have largely superseded magnetic resonance imaging (MRI).

29 Sadomasochism:

(a) Many sadomasochistic practitioners report childhood traumas.
(b) Sadomasochistic behaviours are necessary for orgasm among its practitioners.
(c) Men are more likely than women to assume subservient identities in these behaviours.
(d) Pain is an essential component.
(e) Devotees of sadomasochism have a high pain threshold.

30 Fetishistic behaviours:

(a) Amphetamine misuse can be associated with fetishistic behaviours.
(b) Cocaine misuse can be associated with fetishistic behaviours.
(c) Temporal lobe epilepsy can be associated with fetishistic behaviours.
(d) Fetishistic behaviours occur solely in higher primates.
(e) Fetishistic behaviours occur solely in men.

26  (a) False (p. 117): early in the infection.
    (b) False (p. 117): found in the majority of cases of advanced HIV.
    (c) False (p. 117): more than 50%.
    (d) True (p. 117): caused by opportunistic infections or tumours.
    (e) False (p. 118): much lower – probably 5–15%.

27  (a) True (p. 119).
    (b) True (p. 119).
    (c) False (p. 119): cerebral atrophy and white matter pallor.
    (d) True (p. 119).
    (e) True (p. 119): also leuco-encephalopathy.

28  (a) True (p. 119): cortical atrophy and enlarged ventricles.
    (b) False (p. 119): MRI.
    (c) False (p. 120): lack of correlation.
    (d) True (p. 119): also tumours.
    (e) False (p. 120): instruments of research.

29  (a) False (p. 144).
    (b) False (p. 144): in one study only 15% could achieve orgasm by
        such behaviours alone.
    (c) True (p. 145).
    (d) False (p. 145): it is the illusion of pain.
    (e) False (p. 145): no difference.

30  (a) True (p. 148).
    (b) True (p. 148).
    (c) True (p. 148).
    (d) False (p. 147): also in lower primates.
    (e) False (p. 148): but more men than women.

31   The following are paraphilias:

(a)   Zoophilia.
(b)   Necrophilia.
(c)   Urophilia.
(d)   Apotemnophilia.
(e)   Arachnophilia.


32   The following are true statements in relation to transvestism:

(a)   It typically begins at 15 years of age.
(b)   It sometimes occurs following trauma.
(c)   It is usually not concealed in early childhood.
(d)   Many transvestites continue as fetishists.
(e)   The compulsion to cross-dress is reduced when the person is given the opportunity to express feelings more freely.

31  (a)  True  (p. 150): bestiality.
    (b)  True  (p. 150).
    (c)  True  (p. 151): the use of urine for sexual arousal (coprophilia for faeces).
    (d)  True  (p. 150): sexual arousal by people who are crippled or have amputations.
    (e)  False (p. 150): this is a love of spiders.

32  (a)  False  (p. 161): age 8 or in puberty.
    (b)  True  (p. 161): for example following the loss of a partner.
    (c)  False (p. 161): in secret but without guilt.
    (d)  True  (p. 161).
    (e)  True  (p. 162).

# Psychiatric Genetics

1   The following are true:

(a)   Reciprocal translocations occur when chromosomes of two different pairs exchange segments.

(b)   Robertsonian translocation describes the fusion of two chromosomes at their centromeres.

(c)   Demonstration of the fragile site in fragile X depends upon culturing cells in conditions of thymidine deprivation.

(d)   Messenger RNA is synthesised directly from one strand of DNA.

(e)   'Anticipation' occurs in myotonic dystrophy.


2   Genomic imprinting occurs in:

(a)   Prader–Willi syndrome.

(b)   Angleman syndrome.

(c)   Huntington's chorea.

(d)   Myotonic dystrophy.

(e)   Fragile X syndrome.


3   The following are features of tuberose sclerosis:

(a)   Autosomal recessive inheritance.

(b)   'Tower' skull.

(c)   Deafness.

(d)   Renal cysts.

(e)   Sclerotic brain nodules.


4   The following follow a pattern of autosomal dominant inheritance:

(a)   Laurence Moon Biedl syndrome.

(b)   Treacher Collins syndrome.

(c)   Ataxia telangiectasia.

(d)   Nephrogenic diabetes insipidus.

(e)   Duchenne muscular dystrophy.


5   Fragile X syndrome:

(a)   It is the third commonest genetic cause of mental retardation.

(b)   The fragile site is located at q25.

(c)   Microcephaly is a characteristic clinical feature.

(d)   The molecular basis is related to an heritable sequence of the CTG trinucleotide repeat.

(e)   The expression of fragile X sites is highly correlated with intelligence.

1    (a)  True (p. 7).
     (b)  True (p. 7).
     (c)  True (p. 7).
     (d)  True (p. 9).
     (e)  True (p. 14).

2    (a)  True (p. 14): the expression of a gene or set of genes differs according
          to whether the relevant chromosomes are of maternal or paternal
          origin.
     (b)  True (p. 14).
     (c)  True (p. 14).
     (d)  False.
     (e)  False.

3    (a)  False (p. 70): autosomal dominant.
     (b)  False (p. 70): a feature of Apert's syndrome and Crouzon's syndrome.
     (c)  False (p. 70).
     (d)  True (p. 70).
     (e)  True (p. 70).

4    (a)  False (p. 71): autosomal recessive.
     (b)  True (p. 70).
     (c)  False (p. 71): autosomal recessive.
     (d)  False (p. 71): X-linked.
     (e)  False (p. 71): X-linked.

5    (a)  False (p. 75): it is the second commonest cause, next to Down's
          syndrome.
     (b)  False (p. 75): it is at q27.
     (c)  False (p. 75): macrocephaly.
     (d)  False (p. 76): it is CGG.
     (e)  True (p. 76).

6     Prader–Willi syndrome is a disorder characterised by:

(a)   Deficits in performance tests rather than verbal ability.
(b)   Spasticity.
(c)   Almond-shaped eyes.
(d)   Hypogenitalism.
(e)   A defect at chromosome 15q of maternal origin.

6   (a)  False (p. 80): this is a feature of Turner's syndrome.
    (b)  False (p. 80): hypotonia.
    (c)  True (p. 80).
    (d)  True (p. 81).
    (e)  False (p. 81): it is paternal.

# Child and Adolescent Psychiatry

1 The following are true of a baby's social developmental milestones:
(a) Will smile at its mother within 6 weeks.
(b) Will smile at its mirror image at 5 months.
(c) May show stranger shyness at 6 months.
(d) Waves goodbye at 9 months.
(e) Drinks from a cup at 1 year.

2 The following are true of speech developmental milestones:
(a) Vocalises at 4–6 weeks.
(b) Enjoys vocal play at 5 months.
(c) Has double-syllable sounds at 6 months.
(d) Babbles tunefully at 6 months.
(e) Joins 2 or 3 words in sentences by 18 months.

3 The following are true of motor developmental milestones:
(a) Grasp reflex is absent by 3 months.
(b) 'Mouths' objects at 5 months.
(c) Transfers objects from one hand to another by 5 months.
(d) Has a pincer grasp by 7 months.
(e) Lets go of objects by 10 months.

4 The following vision and hearing developmental milestones are normal:
(a) Turns head to sounds at 6 weeks.
(b) Will localise sound 18 inches lateral to either ear by 4 months.
(c) Will look for toys dropped by 7 months.
(d) Drops toys and watches where they go by 1 year.
(e) Follows dangling toy from side to side at 3 months.

5 The following developmental milestones are normal:
(a) Pulls self to sit at 3 months.
(b) Has a palmar grasp of cube at 6 months.
(c) Babbles 2 or 3 words repeatedly at 9 months.
(d) Understands simple commands at 1 year.
(e) Draws a person at 5 years.

1   (a)  True  (p. 8).
    (b)  True  (p. 8).
    (c)  True  (p. 8).
    (d)  False  (p. 8): 1 year.
    (e)  False  (p. 9): 18 months.

2   (a)  False  (p. 8): 6–8 weeks.
    (b)  True  (p. 8).
    (c)  True  (p. 8).
    (d)  False  (p. 8): 9–10 months.
    (e)  False  (p. 9): 2 years.

3   (a)  True  (p. 8).
    (b)  True  (p. 8).
    (c)  False  (p. 8): 6 months.
    (d)  False  (p. 8): 9–10 months.
    (e)  False  (p. 8): 1 year.

4   (a)  False  (p. 8): 3 months.
    (b)  False  (p. 8): 6 months.
    (c)  False  (p. 8): 9–10 months.
    (d)  True  (p. 8).
    (e)  True  (p. 8).

5   (a)  False  (p. 8): 6 months.
    (b)  True  (p. 8).
    (c)  False  (p. 8): 1 year.
    (d)  True  (p. 8).
    (e)  True  (p. 8): can draw a person on request at 3 years.

6 A 3-year-old child can be expected to have achieved the following developmental milestones:

(a) Goes downstairs one foot per step.
(b) Has imaginary companions.
(c) Dresses and undresses with assistance.
(d) Dry by day.
(e) Gives age.

7 An 18-month-old child can be expected to have achieved the following developmental milestones:

(a) Begins to jump with both feet.
(b) Can throw a ball.
(c) Drink from a cup using both hands.
(d) Builds tower of 6 cubes.
(e) Has parallel play.

8 Sleep in childhood:

(a) The total sleeping time of a newborn baby is 16–17 hours per day.
(b) By 4 months over 80% of babies sleep right through the night.
(c) Only 10% of children at age 1 year are still wakening every night.
(d) 'Transitional objects' may help some children settle at night.
(e) Sleep difficulties are rarer in children aged 2–3 years than in newborn babies.

9 Night terrors:

(a) Usually occur between 2 and 3 years of age.
(b) Occur in stage 3 sleep.
(c) Are often associated with painful events.
(d) Are recalled on awakening.
(e) Are prevented by arousal of the child.

10 Bowel and bladder control:

(a) Voluntary control does not begin until 15–18 months.
(b) Most children are reasonably dry by day at 18 months.
(c) By 2 years 50% are dry at night.
(d) Bowel control is usually acquired before bladder control.
(e) Eneuresis beyond the age of 4 years is considered abnormal.

11 With regard to language development the following are true:

(a) Twins are usually slower to speak than singletons.
(b) Children of higher social class are more advanced in their speech.
(c) Comprehension long precedes the ability to articulate.
(d) Left-handedness is commoner in children with language delay.
(e) Absence of babbling is a pointer to deafness.

6  (a) False (p. 9): two feet per step down and one foot per step upstairs.
   (b) True (p. 9).
   (c) False (p. 9): only undresses with assistance.
   (d) True (p. 9).
   (e) False (p. 9): age 5 years.

7  (a) True (p. 9).
   (b) True (p. 9).
   (c) True (p. 9).
   (d) False (p. 9): 2 years.
   (e) False (p. 9): 2 years.

8  (a) True (p. 10): drops to 13 hours within 6 months.
   (b) False (p. 10): by 6 months.
   (c) True (p. 10).
   (d) True (p. 10).
   (e) False (p. 10): such difficulties are common.

9  (a) False (p. 10): age 3–4 years.
   (b) False (p. 10): stage 4 sleep.
   (c) False (p. 10): not an association.
   (d) False (p. 10): not remembered.
   (e) True (p. 10).

10  (a) True (p. 11).
    (b) True (p. 11).
    (c) True (p. 11): 75% by age 3, 90% by age 5.
    (d) True (p. 11).
    (e) False (p. 11): age 5 for eneuresis and age 4 for encopresis.

11  (a) True (p. 15).
    (b) True (p. 15): children in large families or slums are usually slower
        to speak.
    (c) True (p. 15).
    (d) False (p. 15): although this is controversial, but left-handedness is
        commoner among those with generalised learning difficulties.
    (e) False (p. 15): deaf children babble.

12   The following are true in relation to specific reading retardation:
(a)  Specific reading retardation is when a child's reading age is plus or minus two standard deviations from that expected.
(b)  Its prevalence was 4% among 9–10-year-olds in the Isle of Wight study.
(c)  The male:female ratio is 2:1.
(d)  It is associated with left/right confusion.
(e)  It is associated with visual defects.

13   The following statements regarding stages of psychosocial development are correct:
(a)  Freud's oral stage corresponds with Erikson's stage of autonomy.
(b)  Piaget's sensory motor stage is from 0 to 3 years.
(c)  Kohlberg's pre-conventional morality is from 0 to 9 years.
(d)  Piaget's concrete operational stage corresponds in time with Freud's latency period.
(e)  Freud's phallic phase is from the third to fifth year.

14   Piaget's pre-operational stage has the following features or characteristics:
(a)  Pre-causal logic.
(b)  Authoritarian morality.
(c)  The ability to retain an internalised representation of objects.
(d)  Children at this stage are no longer egocentric.
(e)  Childhood phobias are common in this animistic stage.

15   In Piaget's stage of concrete operations:
(a)  Children lose their animism.
(b)  Children start to use categories.
(c)  Children can anticipate consequences by manipulating mental constructs.
(d)  Painful procedures are seen as punishments.
(e)  Conservation of weight occurs before conservation of number.

16   Kohlberg's moral development:
(a)  Level 1 applies to children up to about 10 years.
(b)  In pre-conventional morality behaviour is guided entirely by internal contingencies.
(c)  Throughout the conventional morality stage a child conforms to avoid others' disapproval.
(d)  In level 3 actions are guided by the principle of a social contract.
(e)  The 'ethical principle orientation' is established in most children at level 3.

12  (a)  False (p. 16): it is 1.5–2 standard deviations *below* that expected.
    (b)  True (p. 16): 10% in the inner-London borough study.
    (c)  False (p. 16): ratio is 3:1.
    (d)  True (p. 16).
    (e)  True (p. 16): also episodic hearing impairment, speech delay, family history of reading difficulties, conduct disorder, large family.

13  (a)  False (p. 18): Freud's oral stage in the first year corresponds with Erikson's trust versus mistrust.
    (b)  False (p. 18): 0–2 years.
    (c)  False (p. 18): 0–7 years.
    (d)  True (p. 8): this roughly corresponds also with Erikson's industry versus inferiority.
    (e)  True (p. 8).

14  (a)  True (p. 20): non-scientific reasoning.
    (b)  True (p. 20).
    (c)  True (p. 20).
    (d)  False (p. 20): are egocentric.
    (e)  True (p. 21): also fears.

15  (a)  True (p. 21).
    (b)  True (p. 21).
    (c)  False (p. 21): formal operational stage.
    (d)  False (p. 21): pre-operational.
    (e)  False (p. 21): the reverse is true, on average at ages 6 and 7, respectively.

16  (a)  False (p. 23): the pre-conventional stage is up to about age 7 years.
    (b)  False (p. 23): it is guided entirely by external contingencies.
    (c)  False (p. 23): at first this is true but it develops into a sense of an externally imposed obligation.
    (d)  True (p. 23).
    (e)  False (p. 24): only 10% in Kohlberg's subjects.

17   The following are true statements in relation to social and emotional development:
(a)   By 6–8 months of age specific attachments develop.
(b)   Stranger anxiety is prominent at 9–12 months.
(c)   Specific attachments of infants are not hierarchical.
(d)   Attachment intensity peaks at 18 months.
(e)   Elaborate fantasies in preschool years are commoner in children with disordered attachments.

18   Genetic factors are a significant contributing factor to the following:
(a)   Tourette's syndrome.
(b)   Childhood depression.
(c)   Childhood schizophrenia.
(d)   Nocturnal enuresis.
(e)   Conduct disorder.

19   The following statements are true:
(a)   There is an inverse relationship between IQ and the prevalence of psychiatric disorders.
(b)   Children with specific reading retardation show higher rates of conduct disorders.
(c)   Children with chronic illness show a two- to threefold increase in psychiatric disorder.
(d)   Children with perceptual difficulties have higher rates of psychiatric disorder.
(e)   Children who experience multiple hospital admissions are at greater risk for later conduct disorder.

20   The following statements are true:
(a)   Children in one-parent families have higher rates of conduct and emotional disorder.
(b)   Children who come from families with four or more children are twice as likely to develop conduct disorder.
(c)   Children with specific learning difficulties have higher rates of conduct disorder.
(d)   Psychiatric morbidity in mothers is associated with conduct disorder.
(e)   The youngest children in a family are more likely to develop conduct disorder than older siblings.

21   The following are correct with reference to axes on ICD–10:
(a)   Developmental disorders are recorded on Axis III.
(b)   The intellectual level is recorded on Axis IV.
(c)   Clinical psychiatric syndrome is recorded on Axis I.
(d)   Axis V denotes associated abnormal psychosocial situation.
(e)   Physical disorders are recorded on Axis II.

17  (a)  True (p. 24).
    (b)  True (p. 24).
    (c)  False (p. 24).
    (d)  True (p. 24): this varies and age 3 years is also noted (see p. 31).
    (e)  False (p. 25): part of normal development.

18  (a)  True (p. 41): familial loading.
    (b)  False (p. 41).
    (c)  True (p. 41).
    (d)  True (p. 42).
    (e)  False (p. 42).

19  (a)  True (p. 42).
    (b)  True (p. 43).
    (c)  True (p. 43).
    (d)  True (p. 43).
    (e)  True (p. 45).

20  (a)  True (p. 46): greater social and economic hardship.
    (b)  True (p. 47).
    (c)  True (p. 43).
    (d)  True (p. 48).
    (e)  False (p. 47): slightly greater risk of school refusal.

21  (a)  False (p. 57): these are on Axis II.
    (b)  False (p. 57): this is on Axis III.
    (c)  True (p. 57).
    (d)  True (p. 57).
    (e)  False (p. 57): these are on Axis IV.

22   The following are true statements:
(a)   Both ICD–10 and DSM–IV use a categorical rather than a dimensional approach.
(b)   Pervasive developmental disorder is coded under Axis II in ICD–10.
(c)   Stuttering is coded under Axis II in ICD–10.
(d)   Tic disorders are classified under Axis III in ICD–10.
(e)   Specific developmental disorders of language are coded under Axis II in ICD–10.

23   Night terrors/sleepwalking:
(a)   Night terrors affect 10% of children.
(b)   Sleepwalking children avoid objects in their path.
(c)   Approximately 50% of children with either sleepwalking or night terrors have a close family relative with a similar history.
(d)   These conditions usually resolve spontaneously within months.
(e)   They are thought to represent a fault in fast-wave sleep.

24   Pica:
(a)   Occurs more frequently in young deprived children.
(b)   Occurs in children with pervasive developmental disorder.
(c)   Is associated with megaloblastic anaemia.
(d)   Is associated with lead poisoning.
(e)   May respond to iron therapy.

25   Infantile autism:
(a)   Is 10 times commoner in boys than girls.
(b)   Does not show social class bias.
(c)   For diagnostic purposes there needs to be evidence of delay or deviant development within the first 3 years.
(d)   Approximately 75% of autistic children do not develop any useful speech.
(e)   Often fail to use anticipatory gestures.

26   Infantile autism is associated with:
(a)   Congenital rubella.
(b)   Cytomegalovirus.
(c)   Phenylketonuria.
(d)   Tuberose sclerosis.
(e)   Neurofibromatosis.

27   Rett's syndrome:
(a)   Occurs only rarely in boys.
(b)   Is characterised by progressive loss of acquired abilities.
(c)   Is characterised by an absence of normal development.
(d)   Is associated with microcephaly at birth.
(e)   Is associated with mild to moderate learning difficulties.

22  (a)  True (p. 57).
    (b)  True (p. 59).
    (c)  False (p. 59): Axis I.
    (d)  False (p. 58): Axis I.
    (e)  True (p. 59).

23  (a)  False (p. 100): approximately 3%.
    (b)  True (p. 100).
    (c)  True (p. 100).
    (d)  True (p. 101).
    (e)  False (p. 100): slow-wave sleep.

24  (a)  True (p. 104).
    (b)  True (p. 104).
    (c)  False (p. 104): iron deficiency.
    (d)  True (p. 104): can lead to lead poisoning.
    (e)  True (p. 104).

25  (a)  False (p. 106): ratio of 3:1 (or 4:1).
    (b)  True (p. 106).
    (c)  True (p. 106).
    (d)  False (p. 106): approximately 50%.
    (e)  True (p. 107).

26  (a)  True (p. 108).
    (b)  True (p. 108).
    (c)  True (p. 108).
    (d)  True (p. 108).
    (e)  True (p. 108): also true for fragile X syndrome.

27  (a)  False (p. 109): described only in girls.
    (b)  True (p. 109).
    (c)  False (p. 109): apparently normal development in the first 1–2 years.
    (d)  False (p. 110): they have a normal head circumference at birth and later deceleration of head growth.
    (e)  False (p. 110): profound learning difficulties.

28   Heller's syndrome:

(a)   Heller's syndrome is also known as childhood disintegrative disorder.
(b)   It occurs in girls only.
(c)   It is characterised by 'normal' development until 2 years of age.
(d)   It is characterised by a profound regression.
(e)   The loss of skills is not necessarily permanent.

29   Asperger's syndrome:

(a)   Intelligence is usually within the mild learning disability range.
(b)   Language prosidy is often peculiar.
(c)   The male:female ratio is about equal.
(d)   Sufferers have normal early language develoment.
(e)   Clumsiness occurs in some children with the syndrome.

30   Reactive attachment disorder:

(a)   Is a probable consequence of severe parental neglect.
(b)   Is a possible marker of disturbed emotional development.
(c)   Must be present before 3 years of age.
(d)   Presents as pervasive disturbances in reciprocal social interactions.
(e)   Is coded in ICD–10 under Axis II, developmental disorders.

31   Emotional disorders:

(a)   It is appropriate for toddlers and preschool children to show separation anxiety disorder.
(b)   Many emotional disorders of early childhood are exaggerations of 'normal development'.
(c)   In the first 3 years specific fears are usually related to imaginary events.
(d)   Sibling rivalry disorders usually emerge when the baby is 6 months old.
(e)   Anxiety and phobic states in children have a variable prognosis.

32   Gender identity disorder:

(a)   Most children by 3 years of age have developed a definite gender identity.
(b)   When gender identity is established it usually remains fixed.
(c)   Prenatal hormones may influence gender identity.
(d)   Gender identity disorder occurs equally in boys and girls.
(e)   Biological factors are probably more important than psychological factors.

33   Common presentations of anxiety disorders in middle childhood include:

(a)   Palpitations.
(b)   Sleeping difficulties.
(c)   Headaches.
(d)   Sweating.
(e)   Depersonalisation.

28  (a)  True (p. 110).
    (b)  False (p. 110): boys and girls.
    (c)  True (p. 110).
    (d)  True (p. 110).
    (e)  True (p. 110): may be followed by a degree of recovery.

29  (a)  False (p. 110): normal range.
    (b)  True (p. 111): staccato or monotonous.
    (c)  False (p. 111): male excess.
    (d)  True (p. 111): relatively normal.
    (e)  True (p. 111).

30  (a)  True (p. 112).
    (b)  True (p. 112).
    (c)  False (p. 112): age 5 years.
    (d)  False (p. 112): not pervasive.
    (e)  False (p. 112): Axis I.

31  (a)  False (p. 117): it is appropriate to show anxiety but not the disorder.
    (b)  True (p. 116).
    (c)  False (p. 117): actual events, the dark, thunder, insects and animals.
    (d)  False (p. 118): usually within 1 month after birth of sibling.
    (e)  False (p. 118): good prognosis.

32  (a)  False (p. 119): age 3–4 years.
    (b)  True (p. 119).
    (c)  False (p. 119): may influence gender-related behaviour.
    (d)  False (p. 120): males more than females.
    (e)  False (p. 120): the reverse is true.

33  (a)  False (p. 124): unlikely.
    (b)  True (p. 125).
    (c)  True (p. 125).
    (d)  False (p. 124): unlikely.
    (e)  False (p. 124): unlikely.

34   Fears and phobias in middle childhood:

(a)   Middle childhood is a time when specific fears lessen.
(b)   Animal phobias are commoner in girls at this age.
(c)   Many require some form of intervention.
(d)   Phobias affect approximately 5% of children.
(e)   Behavioural methods are usually used if phobia is the only symptom.

35   Depression in middle childhood:

(a)   Depression is more common in girls.
(b)   Anhedonia and boredom may be prominent.
(c)   Depression may present as a decline in academic performance.
(d)   Pharmacotherapy plays a major role.
(e)   Most children have a good prognosis.

36   Obsessive–compulsive disorder in middle childhood:

(a)   Obsessive–compulsive disorder is common in middle childhood.
(b)   Onset is often acute.
(c)   Approximately 30% of parents have the disorder.
(d)   Prognosis is worse when obsessional symptoms are part of an affective illness than when there is a 'pure' obsessive–compulsive disorder.
(e)   Those with a shorter history before referral do better than those with long-standing symptoms.

37   Elective mutism:

(a)   A child has little control over this.
(b)   It occurs equally in boys and girls.
(c)   Approximately 75% of children have a history of minor speech problems.
(d)   Minor abnormalities on electroencephalography (EEG) are common.
(e)   80% improve after 5 years.

38   Hysteria in middle childhood:

(a)   Hysteria in middle childhood is very rare.
(b)   Children most commonly present with disorders of gait.
(c)   Symptoms are generally under the child's conscious control.
(d)   Secondary gain is frequently implicated in aetiological theories.
(e)   It is commoner in girls.

39   Recurrent abdominal pain in middle childhood:

(a)   Recurrent abdominal pain with no organic cause occurs in 25% of 5–6-year-olds.
(b)   It frequently accompanies emotional disorders.
(c)   Pain is usually poorly localised.
(d)   It is common in children without obvious psychological difficulties.
(e)   Pain normally lasts 30 minutes or less.

34   (a)   True (p. 127): for example, the dark or animals.
     (b)   True (p. 127).
     (c)   False (p. 128): most tend to improve even if untreated.
     (d)   False (p. 127): 2%.
     (e)   True (p. 127).

35   (a)   False (p. 128): slightly more common in boys.
     (b)   True (p. 128): especially with older children.
     (c)   True (p. 128).
     (d)   False (p. 129): only for severe cases.
     (e)   True (p. 129).

36   (a)   False (p. 132): it is a rare condition, whereas mild obsessions and
           rituals are a normal part of development, especially at this age.
     (b)   False (p. 132): usually insidious.
     (c)   False (p. 132): 5% with the disorder, while two-thirds of parents have
           the trait.
     (d)   False (p. 133): prognosis is better.
     (e)   True (p. 133).

37   (a)   True (p. 133).
     (b)   False (p. 133): more common in girls.
     (c)   False (p. 133): 50%.
     (d)   True (p. 133).
     (e)   False (p. 134): less than 50% have improved after 5 or 10 years.

38   (a)   True (p. 135).
     (b)   True (p. 135): or loss of limb function.
     (c)   False (p. 135).
     (d)   True (p. 135).
     (e)   False (p. 135): equal gender ratio.

39   (a)   True (p. 136).
     (b)   True (p. 136).
     (c)   True (p. 136).
     (d)   True (p. 136).
     (e)   False (p. 136): a few hours.

40   Conduct disorder:

(a)   Features of conduct disorder include substance misuse.
(b)   It is closely related to specific reading retardation.
(c)   Approximately 30% become delinquent adults.
(d)   Overactivity at 3 years is weakly associated with emotional behaviour in middle childhood.
(e)   Children with good peer relationships do better.

41   Stealing in middle childhood:

(a)   About 25% of primary school children steal at least once.
(b)   'Comfort stealing' occurs in well-socialised children.
(c)   Stealing may be followed by lying.
(d)   There may be a history of emotional neglect.
(e)   Stealing is rarely isolated and is usually associated with other antisocial behaviour.

42   Attention deficit hyperactivity disorder:

(a)   The disorder is found in at least 6% of the population.
(b)   It increases with social adversity and declines with age.
(c)   The first line of treatment is stimulant medication.
(d)   Addiction is a problem with long-term stimulant therapy.
(e)   The prognosis is better where the child has 'normal' intelligence.

43   Enuresis:

(a)   Enuresis is defined as occurring after 4 years of age with no organic cause.
(b)   Approximately 10% of children are still wet at night by 5 years.
(c)   It is three times as common in boys.
(d)   It is associated with larger families.
(e)   Most cases will not change without intervention.

44   Tics:

(a)   Tics are a rapid voluntary purposeless movement.
(b)   They tend to involve extremities.
(c)   They affect 20% of children at some stage.
(d)   All forms of tics are commoner in boys.
(e)   Two-thirds of children with tics have EEG abnormalities.

45   Conduct disorder in adolescence:

(a)   Conduct disorder affects 4–10% of adolescents.
(b)   It frequently begins at this age.
(c)   Death of a same-gender parent in the preschool period may be associated with conduct disorder in adolescence.
(d)   A pattern of aggressive behaviour will generally persist into adulthood.
(e)   Stealing in adolescence for sheer pleasure is common.

40  (a)  False (p. 138).
    (b)  True (p. 138).
    (c)  True (p. 139).
    (d)  False (p. 138).
    (e)  True (p. 139).

41  (a)  False (p. 140): approximately 5%.
    (b)  True (p. 140): those who are 'feeling unloved'.
    (c)  True (p. 140).
    (d)  True (p. 140).
    (e)  False (p. 140): there are two types – 'comfort stealing' is commonest in this age group, but the second type is associated with antisocial behaviour, especially in adolescence.

42  (a)  True (p. 141).
    (b)  True (p. 141).
    (c)  False (p. 142): combination of advice and behavioural intervention.
    (d)  False (p. 142).
    (e)  True (p. 142).

43  (a)  False (p. 143): age 5 years.
    (b)  True (p. 143).
    (c)  False (p. 143): twice as common.
    (d)  True (p. 143).
    (e)  False (p. 144): most resolve without formal treatment.

44  (a)  False (p. 145): involuntary.
    (b)  False (p. 146): face, neck and arms.
    (c)  True (p. 146).
    (d)  True (p. 146).
    (e)  True (p. 146): non-specific abnormalities.

45  (a)  True (p. 155).
    (b)  False (p. 155): it frequently begins in middle childhood.
    (c)  True (p. 155).
    (d)  True (p. 157).
    (e)  False (p. 156): usual motive is to obtain money for pursuits.

46   Suicide and deliberate self-harm in adolescence:

(a)   Self-harm is usually premeditated.
(b)   The highest risk of repetition is seen in older females.
(c)   1–2% of those attempting suicide will eventually succeed.
(d)   There is a recurrence rate of approximately 20% within a year following one episode of deliberate self-harm.
(e)   Cutting often has a dysphoric-reducing effect.

47   Anxiety states in adolescence:

(a)   Fear of political events is a common focus.
(b)   School refusal is a prominent symptom in younger adolescents.
(c)   Approximately 50% of sufferers have a family history of phobic or panic disorder.
(d)   Major depression is common as a co-morbid state.
(e)   Exposure to feared situations is recommended in combination with benzodiazepines.

48   Anorexia nervosa:

(a)   The peak prevalence is around 17 years of age.
(b)   The prevalence rate in independent girls' schools is 1 in 100 after 16 years.
(c)   Voluntary starvation of carbohydrate and fat is frequently found.
(d)   Skin-fold thickness is a more accurate long-term measure of nutrition than weight.
(e)   Approximately 50% of anorectic patients make a good recovery.

49   Common features of physically abused children include:

(a)   Pseudo-adult behaviour.
(b)   Poor social interaction.
(c)   Failure to enjoy pleasurable things.
(d)   Low self-esteem.
(e)   Hypervigilance.

50   Known risk factors of child abuse include:

(a)   All social classes.
(b)   Older parents.
(c)   A parent who was abused as a child.
(d)   A parent figure who is biologically unrelated to the child.
(e)   Being a first-born child.

51   Features of the pre-morbid childhood status of schizophrenia include:

(a)   Emotional and behavioural symptoms.
(b)   Schizoid-type personality traits.
(c)   Consistently lower IQs.
(d)   Impoverished family relations.
(e)   Severe shyness.

46   (a)  False (p. 166): usually an impulsive gesture.
     (b)  False (p. 167): older males from larger families.
     (c)  True (p. 167).
     (d)  True (p. 167): 15–25%.
     (e)  True (p. 167).

47   (a)  True (p. 168).
     (b)  True (p. 169).
     (c)  False (p. 169): approximately one-third.
     (d)  True (p. 169).
     (e)  False (pp. 169, 167): exposure through relaxation training and graded
          exposure in imagination.

48   (a)  True (p. 175).
     (b)  True (p. 175).
     (c)  True (p. 176).
     (d)  True (p. 177).
     (e)  True (p. 177): at least as far as weight is concerned.

49   (a)  True (p. 219).
     (b)  True (p. 219).
     (c)  True (p. 219).
     (d)  True (p. 219).
     (e)  True (p. 219).

50   (a)  False (p. 219): usually socially deprived parents.
     (b)  False (p. 219): parental youth and immaturity.
     (c)  True (p. 219).
     (d)  True (p. 219).
     (e)  True (p. 219).

51   (a)  True (p. 283).
     (b)  False (p. 283).
     (c)  False (p. 283): sometimes lower IQ.
     (d)  True (p. 283): but non-specific.
     (e)  False (p. 283).

# Liaison Psychiatry

1    Patients with somatisation disorder have been found to have a frequent family history of:
(a)   Alcohol misuse.
(b)   Antisocial personality.
(c)   Somatisation disorders.
(d)   Affective illness.
(e)   Eating disorders.

2    Patient characteristics associated with increased risk of suicide:
(a)   Younger age.
(b)   Female.
(c)   Being unemployed.
(d)   Living with parents.
(e)   Physical illness.

3    The following are correct in relation to the CAGE questionnaire:
(a)   Subjects are 'CAGE positive' if they answer yes to all four items.
(b)   'Has anyone ever asked you about your drinking habits?' is a CAGE item.
(c)   'Have you ever felt guilty about your drinking?' is a CAGE item.
(d)   'Has your career suffered as a consequence of your drinking?' is a CAGE item.
(e)   'Do you take a drink first thing in the morning?' is a CAGE item.

4    The following are features of opiate withdrawal syndrome:
(a)   Drowsiness.
(b)   Myositis.
(c)   Pinpoint pupils.
(d)   Bradycardia.
(e)   Constipation.

5    The following are true of somatisation disorders:
(a)   ICD–10 requires a minimum of 2 years for the diagnosis of multiple somatisation disorder.
(b)   Patients who receive sickness benefits may remain disabled longer.
(c)   There is consistent evidence that litigation increases the severity of pain.
(d)   Settlement leads to amelioration of symptoms in patients involved in compensation claims.
(e)   Addiction to prescribed drugs is unlikely in chronic somatisers.

1   (a) True (p. 44).
    (b) True (p. 44).
    (c) True (p. 44).
    (d) True (p. 44).
    (e) False (p. 44).

2   (a) False (p. 78): older age.
    (b) False (p. 78): male.
    (c) True (p. 78).
    (d) False (p. 78): living alone.
    (e) True (p. 78).

3   (a) False (p. 87): two or more items determines 'CAGE positive'.
    (b) False (p. 87): 'Have you ever felt annoyed by someone criticising your drinking?' is the item.
    (c) True (p. 87).
    (d) False (p. 87): 'Have you ever tried to cut down on your drinking?' is the CAGE item.
    (e) True (p. 87).

4   (a) False (p. 90): restlessness and insomnia.
    (b) False (p. 90): myalgia.
    (c) False (p. 90): dilated pupils.
    (d) False (p. 90): tachycardia.
    (e) False (p. 90): abdominal pain, vomiting, diarrhoea. Also sweating, piloerection, running nose and eyes.

5   (a) True (p. 112).
    (b) True (p. 112).
    (c) False (p. 112): inconsistent evidence.
    (d) False (p. 112).
    (e) False (p. 113): not uncommon.

6   The following conditions are classified as somatoform disorders in ICD–10:
(a)   Body dysmorphic disorder.
(b)   Neurasthenia.
(c)   Conversion disorders.
(d)   Somatoform autonomic dysfunction.
(e)   Depersonalisation–derealisation disorder.


7   Typical features of a patient with somatisation disorder include:
(a)   Male.
(b)   Age 40–50 years.
(c)   A complicated medical history.
(d)   Holds an invalidity pension.
(e)   Has had a hysterectomy.


8   The following statements are true:
(a)   Patients are likely to cope better with coronary artery disease than with cancer.
(b)   Secretiveness regarding the illness is associated with better psychological adaptation.
(c)   Up to 50% of women fail to adapt to the loss of a breast.
(d)   There is a strong relationship between adverse affects caused by radiotherapy and subsequent psychological morbidity.
(e)   Conditioned nausea and vomiting occur in up to 25% of patients receiving chemotherapy.


9   The following are correct statements:
(a)   People who react to cancer by stoic acceptance survive longer than those who respond by 'denial'.
(b)   The Isle of Wight study found a rate of psychiatric disorder in physically ill 10-year-olds of 13%.
(c)   In the Isle of Wight study, among children with a neurological disorder the rate of psychiatric disorder was almost four times that of the general population.
(d)   If cimetidine is begun after the start of moclobemide treatment it is advisable to reduce the dosage of moclobemide by 50%.
(e)   Most non-steroidal anti-inflammatory agents interact with lithium, resulting in decreased levels of lithium.


10   The following commonly prescribed drugs can precipitate depression:
(a)   Clonidine.
(b)   Metoclopramide.
(c)   Theophylline.
(d)   Indomethacin.
(e)   Nifedipine.

6   (a)  False (p. 115): such cases are classified as a variant of hypochondriacal disorder.
    (b)  False (p. 115): separate category.
    (c)  False (p. 115): grouped with dissociative disorders.
    (d)  True (p. 115).
    (e)  False (p. 115): separate category.

7   (a)  False (p. 119): female.
    (b)  True (p. 119).
    (c)  True (p. 119).
    (d)  True (p. 119).
    (e)  True (p. 119): also on numerous drugs and has spurious physical diagnosis.

8   (a)  True (p. 158): linked to self-blame over cancer.
    (b)  False (p. 160).
    (c)  False (p. 161): up to 25%.
    (d)  True (p. 164).
    (e)  True (p. 163).

9   (a)  False (p. 187).
    (b)  True (p. 195).
    (c)  True (p. 196): the percentage was 24%.
    (d)  True (p. 245): if cimetidine is begun after the start of moclobemide treatment it is advisable to reduce the dosage of moclobemide by 50% and then adjust accordingly.
    (e)  False (pp. 246–247): most non-steroidal anti-inflammatory agents interact with lithium, resulting in an increased level and toxicity.

10  (a)  True (p. 249).
    (b)  True (p. 249).
    (c)  True (p. 249).
    (d)  True (p. 249).
    (e)  True (p. 249).

11 The following commonly prescribed drugs do not precipitate psychosis:
(a) Pergolide.
(b) Clonidine.
(c) Hydrocortisone.
(d) Ephedrine.
(e) Digoxin.

11  (a)  False (p. 249).
    (b)  False (p. 249).
    (c)  False (p. 249).
    (d)  False (p. 249).
    (e)  False (p. 249).

# General Adult Psychiatry

1   The following are correct statements:
(a)   Depressed mood is the commonest symptom to be found in depressive disorders.
(b)   Anxiety is one of the commonest symptoms in depressive disorders.
(c)   Agitation is marked anxiety combined with excessive motor activity.
(d)   Anhedonia is the second most common symptom in depressive disorders.
(e)   Guilt is present in 75% of people with depression.

2   The following delusions are regarded as mood incongruent in depressive disorders:
(a)   Delusions of guilt.
(b)   Delusions of poverty.
(c)   Hypochondriacal delusions.
(d)   Delusions of catastrophe.
(e)   Nihilistic delusions.

3   Depersonalisation occurs:
(a)   As a primary phenomenon.
(b)   Following sensory deprivation.
(c)   In temporal lobe epilepsy.
(d)   In phobic anxiety disorders.
(e)   In generalised anxiety disorders.

4   Derealisation includes the following:
(a)   Perception of the environment as soulless.
(b)   Impressions of mystery.
(c)   Loss of vivid image recall.
(d)   Changes in experience of time.
(e)   Perception of surroundings lacking colour.

5   The following statements are true:
(a)   Derealisation is a belief.
(b)   Insight into the abnormal nature of derealisation is absent.
(c)   Depersonalisation can be viewed as a diagnostic sign of depression.
(d)   Depersonalisation is categorised as depersonalisation–derealisation syndrome in ICD–10.
(e)   Depersonalisation is a common symptom of depression.

1    (a)  True  (p. 3).
     (b)  True  (p. 4).
     (c)  True  (p. 4).
     (d)  True  (p. 6).
     (e)  True  (p. 11): to some degree.

2    (a)  False  (p. 15).
     (b)  False  (p. 15).
     (c)  False  (p. 15).
     (d)  False  (p. 15).
     (e)  False  (p. 15).

     Note. These are mood-congruent delusions.

3    (a)  True  (p. 16).
     (b)  True  (p. 16).
     (c)  True  (p. 16).
     (d)  True  (p. 16).
     (e)  True  (p. 16).

     Note. It occurs also in depression, schizophrenia, organic disorders and healthy persons under stress.

4    (a)  True  (p. 16).
     (b)  True  (p. 16).
     (c)  True  (p. 16).
     (d)  True  (p. 16).
     (e)  True  (p. 16).

5    (a)  False  (p. 16): it is an experience, not a belief.
     (b)  False  (p. 16): insight is retained.
     (c)  False  (p. 16).
     (d)  True  (p. 16).
     (e)  False  (p. 15).

6    Obsessive–compulsive phenomena have the following features:

(a)   Obsessive–compulsive symptoms occur in 40% of depressive episodes.
(b)   Many of those who gain obsessions during a depressive episode fail to lose them on recovery.
(c)   In time the experience of conscious resistance may fade.
(d)   It is not classified as an obsession if a patient rechecks that a door is locked unless the patient can remember locking the door.
(e)   The obsessional nature of aggressive thoughts is usually protective against harmful actions.

7    The following are true statements:

(a)   Most studies show that, compared with unipolar disorders, bipolar disorders show an earlier age of onset with more frequent and shorter episodes.
(b)   Unipolar depression is twice as common in women than in men.
(c)   The incidence of bipolar disorders is equal between the genders.
(d)   Combined rates of unipolar and bipolar disorders found in first-degree relatives of bipolar probands are significantly higher than those found in first-degree relatives of unipolar probands.
(e)   Bipolar probands show increased risks of bipolar disorders alone in first-degree relatives.

8    Seasonal affective disorder:

(a)   Carbohydrate craving is a feature.
(b)   Untreated episodes usually resolve by springtime.
(c)   Over 50% of sufferers report a history of affective disorders in at least one first-degree relative.
(d)   Most meet the criteria only for unipolar disorders.
(e)   Recommended treatment is exposure to light of 2500 lux for 4 hours per day.

9    The following are observer rating scales for measuring the severity of depression:

(a)   Hamilton Rating Scale for Depression (Hamilton Depression Rating Scale).
(b)   Montgomery–Åsberg Depression Rating Scale.
(c)   Beck Depression Inventory.
(d)   Zung Depression Scale.
(e)   Leeds Scale.

10   The following are true regarding recovery from depressive disorders:

(a)   Recovery is faster in melancholic episodes.
(b)   Recovery is faster in unipolar episodes.
(c)   High neuroticism scores on the Eysenck Personality Inventory are associated with a slower recovery.
(d)   Hallucinations predict a slower recovery.
(e)   Mood-incongruent features have been shown to predict a slower recovery.

6   (a)  False (p. 17): 20–35%.
    (b)  False (p. 17): this occurs in a few.
    (c)  True (p. 17).
    (d)  True (p. 17).
    (e)  True (p. 17).

7   (a)  True (p. 26).
    (b)  True (p. 26).
    (c)  True (p. 26).
    (d)  True (p. 26).
    (e)  True (p. 26): whereas unipolar probands do not.

8   (a)  True (p. 33): also increased appetite, overeating and hypersomnia.
    (b)  False (p. 33).
    (c)  True (p. 33).
    (d)  True (p. 33).
    (e)  False (p. 34): 2 hours a day. Morning treatment may be better and exposure to the patient's eyes is important.

9   (a)  True (p. 36).
    (b)  True (p. 36).
    (c)  False (p. 37): self-rated.
    (d)  False (p. 37): self-rated
    (e)  False (p. 37): self-rated.

10  (a)  True (p. 40).
    (b)  True (p. 40).
    (c)  True (p. 40).
    (d)  True (p. 40).
    (e)  True (p. 40): as have hypochondriacal symptoms and secondary depression.

11 Predictors of a switch from a depressive to a bipolar episode include:
(a) Early age of onset.
(b) Family history of bipolar disorders.
(c) Retardation.
(d) Hypersomnia.
(e) Occurrence in the year after childbirth.

12 The following are true of bipolar affective disorder:
(a) ICD–10 specifies a single episode of mania or mixed disorder as the minimum for bipolar affective disorder.
(b) Mania occurs with a decreasing frequency in persons with learning disability.
(c) Mania can be measured by Young's observer-rated scale.
(d) The peak age of first hospitalisation is in the late teens.
(e) The episode duration tends to be stable throughout the course of the illness.

13 With regard to rapid cycling the following are true:
(a) Rapid cycling is defined as three or more affective episodes in 1 year.
(b) It is equally common in men and women.
(c) It is more common later in the course of an illness.
(d) Antidepressants can increase the frequency of rapid cycling.
(e) An association has been found with clinical or sub-clinical hypothyroidism.

14 The following statements regarding relapse of bipolar affective disorder are true:
(a) The first episode is more likely to be triggered by life events than are later episodes.
(b) Flying overnight from east to west is more likely to lead to mania than travel in the opposite direction.
(c) Sleep deprivation may trigger a manic episode.
(d) Increased life events in the previous month may trigger mania.
(e) Insomnia may trigger a manic episode.

15 The following are true of lithium:
(a) Patients in a rapid-cycling phase tend not to respond to lithium.
(b) Lithium has a variable plasma half-life of 7–20 hours.
(c) Lithium enhances production of cyclic adenosine monophosphate (cAMP).
(d) It blocks the development of dopamine supersensitivity that normally occurs with antipsychotic drugs.
(e) Goitre and hypothyroidism as side-effects of lithium are due in part to its interference with the action of thyroid-stimulating hormone (TSH) at its receptors in the thyroid.

11  (a)  True (p. 42).
    (b)  True (p. 42).
    (c)  True (p. 42).
    (d)  True (p. 42).
    (e)  True (p. 42).

    Note. Also true for hypomania precipitated by antidepressants, melancholia, and delusions/hallucinations. One in ten of those who begin with a depressive episode go on to develop an episode of mania. The likelihood of a switch drops after the third episode of depression.

12  (a)  False (p. 59): two separate episodes, one of which has been hypomania, mania or mixed.
    (b)  False (p. 60): it occurs with the same frequency.
    (c)  True (p. 60): also scales by Beigel and Blackburn.
    (d)  True (p. 60): the median is in the mid-20s and mean age of first hospitalisation about 26 years.
    (e)  True (p. 61): but onset may become more rapid in later episodes.

13  (a)  False (p. 61): four or more.
    (b)  False (p. 61): it is commoner in women.
    (c)  True (p. 61).
    (d)  True (p. 61): withdrawal of antidepressants can restore 'normal' cycling.
    (e)  True (pp. 61–62): although a causal relationship has not been proved.

14  (a)  True (p. 63): probably in keeping with the process of 'kindling'.
    (b)  False (p. 63): the opposite is true, that is from west to east.
    (c)  True (p. 63).
    (d)  True (p. 63).
    (e)  True (p. 63).

15  (a)  True (p. 70).
    (b)  True (p. 70): longer in elderly and physically unwell.
    (c)  False (p. 71): it inhibits cAMP.
    (d)  True (p. 72).
    (e)  True (p. 71).

16 Lithium's side-effects include:
(a) Increased TSH levels occur in one in four patients.
(b) Thyroid enlargement develops in about 5%.
(c) Polyuria and excessive thirst with polydipsia occurs in one-third.
(d) Fine tremor of the hands occurs in one in four.
(e) Hair loss occurs in about 5%.

17 Lithium has the following laboratory effects:
(a) Increases parathyroid hormone.
(b) Decreases calcium.
(c) Increases TSH.
(d) Decreases glucose tolerance.
(e) Decreases angiotensin levels.

18 The following are features of mild lithium toxicity:
(a) Diarrhoea.
(b) Severe fine tremor.
(c) Vomiting.
(d) Disorientation.
(e) Twitching.

19 The side-effects of carbamazepine include:
(a) A macupapular itchy rash within 2 weeks in up to 10% of patients.
(b) Low white cell counts.
(c) Hyponatraemia due to inhibition of antidiuretic hormone (ADH).
(d) Lowers its own blood levels by liver enzyme induction.
(e) Lowered thyroid hormone metabolism.

20 Regarding prophylaxis of bipolar disorder the following are true:
(a) Maintenance treatment should be instituted after the first major episode.
(b) A family history of bipolar affective disorder is a strong predictor of prophylactic efficacy of lithium.
(c) Studies have indicated that blood levels lower than those formerly used are sufficient for prophylaxis.
(d) Studies indicate a 50% recurrence of mania within 6 months following lithium discontinuation.
(e) Memory impairment is often quoted as a reason for non-adherence to lithium.

21 Factors which predict a good response to lithium prophylaxis in bipolar affective disorder include:
(a) Family history of bipolar affective disorder.
(b) Neurological signs.
(c) Patients whose first episode was depressive.
(d) Rapid cycling of illness.
(e) A good response to lithium in acute mania.

16 (a) True (p. 72).
   (b) True (p. 72): clinical hypothyroidism in 5–10%.
   (c) True (p. 72): usually reversible but not always, especially after long-term treatment.
   (d) True (p. 73).
   (e) True (p. 74): also altered texture of hair.

17 (a) True (p. 74): mild increase.
   (b) False (p. 74): mild increase.
   (c) True (p. 72).
   (d) False (p. 74): increase.
   (e) False (p. 74): it increases angiotensin levels and antagonises aldosterone.

18 (a) True (p. 77): also nausea.
   (b) True (p. 77): also poor concentration.
   (c) False (p. 77): feature of moderate or severe toxicity.
   (d) False (p. 77): feature of moderate toxicity.
   (e) False (p. 77): feature of severe toxicity.

19 (a) True (pp. 78–79): and requires cessation of drug.
   (b) True (p. 79).
   (c) False (p. 79): potentiation of ADH.
   (d) True (p. 79).
   (e) False (p. 79): increased thyroid hormone metabolism.

20 (a) False (p. 81): there is a lot of controversy as to whether maintenance should be started after the first episode or not. In practice treatment is started following the second episode, especially if the interval between episodes is less than 5 years. Consider maintenance treatment after a first episode if there is severe disruptive sudden onset or suicidal risk, or if the episode was not precipitated by external factors.
   (b) True (p. 81).
   (c) True (p. 82).
   (d) True (p. 84).
   (e) True (p. 85): also excessive thirst, polyuria, tremor, weight gain and hair loss.

21 (a) True (p. 81).
   (b) False (p. 81).
   (c) False (p. 81): those whose first episode was manic.
   (d) False (p. 81).
   (e) True (p. 81): this is assumed though unproven.

22   The following statements are incorrect:

(a)   Lithium prophylaxis has an average failure rate of approximately 40%.
(b)   Carbamazepine is as effective in rapid-cycling disorders as in other bipolar affective disorders.
(c)   There may be partial loss of efficacy by the third year of treatment with carbamazepine.
(d)   The combination of lithium and carbamazepine produces fewer neurological problems than lithium alone.
(e)   Valproate appears to be more effective for mania than for depression.

23   The ECA (Epidemiologic Catchment Area) study made the following findings:

(a)   The annual prevalence rate for bipolar affective disorder was 1%.
(b)   The mean age of first onset was 28 years for bipolar affective disorder.
(c)   No significant gender difference was found in the estimated rates of bipolar affective disorder.
(d)   The annual incidence rate for major depression was 6%.
(e)   The overall female:male ratio for dysthymia was 2:1.

24   The following are true:

(a)   The significant gender differences in unipolar disorders are consistent across cultures.
(b)   Non-parous females have a lower rate of first admission for affective disorders than males.
(c)   'Never married subjects' have a low rate of depression.
(d)   There is minimal evidence of racial or ethnic differences in the prevalence of depression.
(e)   There is evidence that areas in transition from a rural to a more industrialised environment show particularly high morbidity rates.

25   Risks of affective disorder:

(a)   The risk of developing bipolar illness in first-degree relatives of bipolar probands is approximately 7%.
(b)   First-degree relatives of unipolar probands have a risk for bipolar illness equal to that of the general population.
(c)   The morbid risk of unipolar illness in first-degree relatives of bipolar probands is over 10%.
(d)   The combined rates for affective disorder are higher in relatives of bipolar probands than in relatives of unipolar probands.
(e)   There is an increased risk in relatives of early-onset probands of both unipolar and bipolar illness.

22  (a)  False (p. 86).
    (b)  False (p. 86).
    (c)  False (p. 86).
    (d)  False (p. 88).
    (e)  False (p. 87).
         Note the negative stem.


23  (a)  True (p. 104): lifetime prevalence is 1.2%.
    (b)  False (p. 104): mean age of onset is 21 years.
    (c)  True (p. 104).
    (d)  False (p. 104): the annual prevalence was 2.7%; the lifetime
         prevalence was 4.4%; the annual incidence was 1.8%.
    (e)  True (p. 104).


24  (a)  True (p. 106): also persistent over time.
    (b)  True (p. 106).
    (c)  True (p. 106).
    (d)  True (p. 107): correcting for socio-economic and educational
         variables.
    (e)  True (p. 107): there is some evidence.


25  (a)  True (p. 108).
    (b)  True (p. 108): 0.7%.
    (c)  True (p. 108): 11.5%.
    (d)  True (p. 108).
    (e)  True (p. 109).

26 The following are true:

(a) Low 5-HIAA levels in the cerebrospinal fluid (CSF) are a marker for depression.

(b) Urinary 3-methoxy-4-hydroxy-phenyl glycol (MHPG) is derived mostly from the brain.

(c) Approximately two-thirds of patients with depression show blunting of the TSH response to TRH.

(d) Thyroid autoantibodies are found in 15% of patients with affective disorders.

(e) Elevated cortisol secretion and dexamethasone non-suppression in depression are associated with a poor prognosis.


27 In the cognitive model of depression the following are correct:

(a) The central issue of the 'learned helplessness' hypothesis is that rewards are non-contingent with actions.

(b) The 'depression-prone' individual possesses a maladaptive attributional style.

(c) The 'hopelessness' model requires matching of a stressor with the attributional style relating to the specific domain of functioning.

(d) Beck's cognitive triad includes negative thoughts about the self, the world and past experiences.

(e) Negative cognitions are sustained through biases in information processing.


28 The following are correct statements:

(a) The prevalence of depression in 'never married' subjects is closest to that of continuously married subjects.

(b) Of the vulnerability/protective factors the role of a confidant in reducing depression is the most robust.

(c) The 'buffer' theory suggests that the lack of social support directly predisposes to depression.

(d) The 'main effect' hypothesis suggests that the presence of social support reduces the risk of depression by modifying the impact of adversity.

(e) Life events during the course of treatment are unlikely to affect depressive symptoms greatly.


29 Tricyclic antidepressants have the following properties:

(a) Because of first-pass metabolism only 50% of an orally administered dose reaches the systemic circulation.

(b) Alcohol has a triphasic effect on the first-pass metabolism of tricyclic antidepressants.

(c) The anticholinergic effect of tricyclic antidepressants explains how they may delay their own absorption.

(d) Secondary amines are more rapidly absorbed than tertiary amines.

(e) The main rate-limiting step in the elimination of tricyclic antidepressants is the biotransformation mediated by hepatic cytochrome P450.

26  (a)  False (p. 115): a marker for impulsivity but not depression.
    (b)  False (p. 113): only 30% is derived from the brain.
    (c)  False (p. 118): one-third. A smaller percentage show an exaggerated response.
    (d)  True (p. 118): also basal TSH is elevated in approximately 15%.
    (e)  True (p. 118): also associated with cognitive failure but are not indications of successful drug treatment.

27  (a)  True (p. 125).
    (b)  True (p. 125).
    (c)  True (p. 126).
    (d)  False (p. 126): Beck's triad related to the self, the world and the future.
    (e)  True (p. 126): information processing biases are systematic errors in thinking such as overgeneralisation and selective abstraction.

28  (a)  True (p. 129).
    (b)  True (p. 129).
    (c)  False (p. 130): the buffer theory suggests that the presence of social support reduces the risk of depression by modifying the effect of adversity.
    (d)  False (p. 130): the main effect hypothesis suggests that the lack of social support directly predisposes to depression.
    (e)  False (p. 135): they may lead to an exacerbation.

29  (a)  True (p. 156).
    (b)  True (p. 157): acute alcohol ingestion can substantially impair first-pass metabolism and so may double or triple the amount of drug reaching the circulation.
    (c)  True (p. 157).
    (d)  False (p. 158): the reverse is true.
    (e)  True (p. 158).

30   The following statements are correct regarding tricyclic anti-depressants:
(a)   Tricyclic antidepressants reach a steady state in approximately 5 days.
(b)   Smoking can decrease tricyclic antidepressant metabolism by enzyme induction.
(c)   Methylphenidate may lower the antidepressant effect of tricyclic anti-depressants.
(d)   Tricyclic antidepressants inhibit the neuronal uptake of clonidine.
(e)   Near complete washout of the drug will take approximately 5 days when discontinued.

31   The following statements concerning tricyclic antidepressants are correct:
(a)   Amitriptyline's metabolite nortriptyline is less noradrenergic.
(b)   Clomipramine can be given intramuscularly.
(c)   Sertraline has a higher serotonin (5-hydroxytryptamine; 5-HT) selectivity than clomipramine.
(d)   Lofepramine is safer than other tricyclics in overdose.
(e)   Desipramine has weak dopamine-blocking activity.

32   The following are true statements:
(a)   Mianserin does not block reuptake of serotonin, noradrenaline or dopamine.
(b)   Maprotiline is particularly prone to cause convulsions.
(c)   Priapism with trazadone has an incidence of 1 in 10 000 males.
(d)   Nefazodone has 5-HT$_{2A}$ agonist activity.
(e)   Venlafaxine has little affinity for muscarinic and noradrenergic receptors.

33   The ophthalmic effects of tricyclic antidepressants include:
(a)   Cycloplegia.
(b)   Presbyopia.
(c)   Sluggish pupillary reaction to light.
(d)   Meiosis.
(e)   Nystagmus.

34   The anticholinergic effects of tricyclic antidepressants may explain the following:
(a)   Faecal impaction.
(b)   Stomatitis.
(c)   Memory impairment.
(d)   Delusional states.
(e)   Fine tremor.

30   (a)   True  (p. 159): assuming a half-life of approximately 24 hours (i.e. this is five times the half-life).
     (b)   False  (p. 160): it can increase tricyclic antidepressant metabolism.
     (c)   False  (p. 160): it enhances because it inhibits tricyclic antidepressant metabolism.
     (d)   True  (p. 160).
     (e)   True  (p. 159).

31   (a)   False  (p. 161): it is more noradrenergic.
     (b)   True  (p. 161).
     (c)   False  (p. 161).
     (d)   True  (p. 163).
     (e)   False  (p. 163): amoxapine has weak dopamine-blocking activity, not desipramine.

32   (a)   True  (p. 164): because mianserin, a tetracyclic, blocks presynaptic alpha$_2$ adrenoceptors.
     (b)   True  (p. 164).
     (c)   False  (p. 165): it is 1 in 6000.
     (d)   False  (p. 165): antagonistic.
     (e)   False  (p. 166): has little affinity for muscarinic, histaminic or alpha$_1$ adrenergic receptors; it is a serotonin and noradrenaline reuptake inhibitor.

33   (a)   True  (p. 167): paresis of ciliary muscle.
     (b)   True  (p. 167): disturbed near vision.
     (c)   True  (p. 167).
     (d)   False  (p. 167): mydriasis.
     (e)   False  (p. 167).

34   (a)   True  (p. 168): and paralytic ileus.
     (b)   True  (p. 167): dry mouth and dental caries.
     (c)   True  (p. 168).
     (d)   True  (p. 168): confusional states.
     (e)   False  (p. 168): unknown mechanism.

35   The cardiovascular effects of tricyclic antidepressants include:

(a)   The most common side-effect is tachycardia.
(b)   They cause a reduction of conduction time in the bundle of His.
(c)   An increase in the PR interval and T-wave amplitude.
(d)   QRS duration and tricyclic antidepressant plasma concentration are weakly correlated following overdose.
(e)   Tricyclic antidepressants have a quinidine-like effect due to the inhibition of sodium–potassium adenosine triphosphatase (ATPase).

36   The side-effects of tricyclic antidepressants:

(a)   Carbohydrate craving with a preference for sweet foods is commonly reported.
(b)   Urticarial rashes are the most common skin reaction.
(c)   Hyponatraemia is rare.
(d)   Impaired liver function occurs in 5%.
(e)   Galactorrhoea is rare.

37   The features of selective serotonin reuptake inhibitors (SSRIs) include:

(a)   Greater than 90% of orally administered dose reaches systemic circulation.
(b)   Fluoxetine inhibits its own metabolism.
(c)   Paroxetine's pharmacokinetics are non-linear.
(d)   SSRI metabolites are mainly excreted in faeces.
(e)   A minimum of 6 weeks should be allowed before an SSRI is started after treatment with a monoamine oxidase inhibitor (MAOI).

38   Further features of SSRIs include:

(a)   Citalopram is the most potent inhibitor of serotonin reuptake.
(b)   Citalopram is a strong inhibitor of cytochrome P450.
(c)   A threefold rise in plasma theophylline levels occurs following administration of fluvoxamine.
(d)   Sertraline clearance is reduced during co-administration with cimetidine.
(e)   Inhibition of cytochrome P450 is reversed within a week of stopping paroxetine.

39   The main clinical features of the serotonin syndrome are:

(a)   Restlessness.
(b)   Confusion.
(c)   Myoclonus.
(d)   Hyper-reflexia.
(e)   Diaphoresis.

35   (a)  False (p. 170): postural hypotension.
     (b)  False (p. 170): prolongation.
     (c)  False (p. 171): an increase in the PR interval, QRS and QT and a
          decrease in T-wave amplitude.
     (d)  False (p. 171): strongly correlated.
     (e)  True (p. 170).

36   (a)  True (p. 172).
     (b)  False (p. 172): eczematous.
     (c)  True (p. 172): inappropriate ADH secretion.
     (d)  False (p. 172): approximately 1%.
     (e)  True (p. 172).

37   (a)  True (p. 174).
     (b)  True (p. 174): also true of paroxetine.
     (c)  True (p. 174).
     (d)  False (p. 176): they are excreted in urine.
     (e)  False (p. 178): 2 weeks.

38   (a)  False (p. 179): although citalopram is the most serotonin selective of
          the SSRIs.
     (b)  False (p. 179): it has weak inhibition.
     (c)  True (p. 180).
     (d)  True (p. 182).
     (e)  True (p. 181).

39   (a)  True (p. 184).
     (b)  True (p. 184).
     (c)  True (p. 184).
     (d)  True (p. 184).
     (e)  True (p. 184).

       Note. Also shivering, tremor, hypomania, incoordination and diarrhoea.

40 MAOIs have the following properties:
(a) All MAOIs are rapidly absorbed.
(b) Anticholinergic adverse reactions are less than with tricyclic antidepressants.
(c) The postural component of hypotension is less than with tricyclic antidepressants.
(d) The effects of antidiabetic agents may be enhanced.
(e) Tyramine-rich foods should be avoided for 4 weeks after the drugs have been stopped.

41 Predictors of a good response to electroconvulsive therapy (ECT) include:
(a) Hypochondriacal symptoms.
(b) Fluctuating course.
(c) Premorbid personality problems.
(d) Depressive delusions.
(e) Biological symptoms.

42 ECT in schizophrenia:
(a) ECT is particularly effective in individuals with delusions of passivity.
(b) Premorbid schizoid personality is a predictor of a good response to ECT.
(c) Perplexity is a predictor of a good response to ECT.
(d) ECT is particularly effective in individuals with delusional mood.
(e) ECT has no place in the management of symptoms of social incongruence associated with chronic schizophrenia.

43 The following factors lower the seizure threshold in ECT:
(a) Male gender.
(b) Lignocaine.
(c) Old age.
(d) Bilateral ECT.
(e) Multiple seizures over the past few weeks.

44 The following factors increase the seizure threshold in ECT:
(a) Reserpine.
(b) Sensory stimulation.
(c) Young.
(d) Female gender.
(e) Benzodiazepines.

45 The following factors prolong the duration of seizure in ECT:
(a) Youth.
(b) Low initial seizure threshold.
(c) Moderate supra-threshold stimulus.
(d) Hypo-oxygenation.
(e) Muscle relaxation.

40　(a)　True　(p. 185).
　　(b)　True　(pp. 186–187).
　　(c)　True　(p. 187): both supine and erect blood pressures are lowered, so the postural component is less.
　　(d)　True　(p. 188).
　　(e)　False　(p. 188): 2 weeks.

41　(a)　False　(p. 221).
　　(b)　False　(p. 221).
　　(c)　True　(p. 221).
　　(d)　True　(p. 221).
　　(e)　True　(p. 221).

42　(a)　True　(p. 222).
　　(b)　False　(p. 222): controversial.
　　(c)　True　(p. 222).
　　(d)　True　(p. 222).
　　(e)　True　(p. 223).

43　(a)　False　(p. 230): raises seizure threshold.
　　(b)　False　(p. 230): raises seizure threshold.
　　(c)　False　(p. 230): raises seizure threshold.
　　(d)　False　(p. 230).
　　(e)　False　(p. 230).

44　(a)　False　(p. 230).
　　(b)　False　(p. 230).
　　(c)　False　(p. 230).
　　(d)　False　(p. 230).
　　(e)　True　(p. 230).

45　(a)　True　(p. 230).
　　(b)　True　(p. 230).
　　(c)　True　(p. 230).
　　(d)　False　(p. 230): shorter duration and *vice versa*.
　　(e)　True　(p. 230).

46 The following cognitive techniques are used in cognitive therapy:

(a) Labelling distortions.
(b) Graded task assignment.
(c) Mastery and pleasure ratings.
(d) Activity scheduling.
(e) Decatastrophising.


47 The following behavioural techniques are used in cognitive therapy:

(a) Relapse prevention.
(b) Challenging assumptions.
(c) Reality testing.
(d) Search for alternatives.
(e) Activity scheduling.


48 Interpersonal psychotherapy has the following components:

(a) It is a brief weekly treatment over 6 months.
(b) It is a here-and-now therapy.
(c) Childhood experiences are a focus of attention.
(d) The therapist reviews all the patient's symptoms.
(e) It focuses mainly on roles within the nuclear and extended family.


49 The following are Schneider's first-rank symptoms:

(a) Third-person auditory hallucination.
(b) *Echo de la pensée.*
(c) Thought blocking.
(d) Delusional perception.
(e) Somatic passivity.


50 Disorders of the form of thought in schizophrenia include:

(a) Blocking.
(b) Decreased speech amount.
(c) Asyndetic thought.
(d) Idiosyncratic logic.
(e) Metonyms.


51 The assessment of cognitive impairment incorporates:

(a) Word-generation task testing executive functioning.
(b) Wisconsin Card-Sorting Test to detect attentional impairment.
(c) The Stroop Task to test selective attention.
(d) The continuous performance test assessing vigilance.
(e) Ability to change strategies in response to change in task demands to test executive functioning.

46  (a)  True (p. 247).
    (b)  False (p. 247): it is a behavioural technique.
    (c)  False (p. 247): behavioural technique.
    (d)  False (p. 247): behavioural technique.
    (e)  True (p. 247).

47  (a)  False (p. 247): it is a preventive strategy.
    (b)  False (p. 247): preventive strategy.
    (c)  False (p. 247): cognitive approach.
    (d)  False (p. 247): cognitive technique.
    (e)  True (p. 247).

48  (a)  False (p. 252): over 12–16 weeks.
    (b)  True (p. 253).
    (c)  False (p. 253): it focuses on current relationships.
    (d)  True (p. 253).
    (e)  False (p. 253): also work, friendship and community.

49  (a)  True (p. 276).
    (b)  True (p. 276): the experience of hearing one's own thoughts aloud.
    (c)  False (p. 277).
    (d)  True (p. 278).
    (e)  True (p. 278).

    Note. Schneider's first-rank symptoms are: voices commenting, voices arguing
    or discussing, audible thoughts, thought broadcasting, thought withdrawal,
    thought insertion, made will, made acts, made affects, somatic passivity and
    delusional perception.

50  (a)  False (p. 284): a disorder of flow.
    (b)  False (p. 284): a disorder of flow.
    (c)  True (p. 284): derailment.
    (d)  True (p. 284).
    (e)  True (p. 284): word approximations.

51  (a)  True (p. 293).
    (b)  False (p. 294): it tests executive functioning.
    (c)  True (p. 294).
    (d)  True (p. 294): it tests the ability to sustain attention.
    (e)  True (pp. 293–294).

52 Factors associated with poor prognosis in schizophrenia include:
(a) Positive family history of affective disorder.
(b) Marked mood disturbance at onset.
(c) Female gender.
(d) Less developed countries.
(e) Enlarged ventricles.

53 The Scale for the Assessment of Negative Symptoms (SANS) includes:
(a) Anhedonia.
(b) Attentional impairment.
(c) Alogia.
(d) Avolition.
(e) Affective flattening.

54 The ICD–10 criteria for schizophrenia include:
(a) 2 weeks' duration of symptoms.
(b) Schizophrenic symptoms must postdate mood disturbance when present.
(c) Minimum presence of two very clear symptoms.
(d) Schizophrenia should not be diagnosed in the presence of overt brain disease.
(e) Any prodromal non-psychotic phase should not be included in the duration criteria.

55 The following epidemiological features of schizophrenia are true:
(a) Incidence is evenly distributed around the world.
(b) Sufferers are more likely to be born in cities.
(c) Immigrants tend to have a higher risk than the general population of their adopted but not native country.
(d) There is an excess of summer births.
(e) There is poor supportive evidence for the social drift hypothesis.

56 In untreated schizophrenia the following brain structures are reduced:
(a) Corpus striatum.
(b) Right temporal lobe.
(c) Temporal horn of left ventricle.
(d) Reduced grey and white matter volume of hippocampus.
(e) Ventricular:brain ratio.

57 The Camberwell Family Interview has the following features:
(a) It is a structured standardised interview.
(b) Ratings are made from audio-tapes.
(c) Scorings are based on content.
(d) Ratings are made of emotional overinvolvement.
(e) Warmth and positive comments are excluded.

52  (a)  False (p. 303): good prognosis.
    (b)  False (p. 303): good prognosis.
    (c)  False (p. 303): good prognosis.
    (d)  False (p. 303): good prognosis.
    (e)  True (p. 303).

53  (a)  True (p. 308).
    (b)  True (p. 308).
    (c)  True (p. 308).
    (d)  True (p. 308).
    (e)  True (p. 308).

54  (a)  False (p. 313): 1 month.
    (b)  False (p. 313): antedate.
    (c)  False (p. 313): one very clear symptom and usually two or more if
         less clear cut.
    (d)  True (p. 313): or p. 89 of ICD–10.
    (e)  True (p. 88 of ICD–10).

55  (a)  True (p. 323).
    (b)  True (p. 325).
    (c)  False (p. 325): both native and adopted countries.
    (d)  False (p. 327): winter and spring births.
    (e)  True (p. 325).

56  (a)  True (p. 344): but increased with long-term neuroleptic treatment.
    (b)  False (p. 345): left temporal lobe.
    (c)  False (p. 345): increased.
    (d)  True (p. 344).
    (e)  False (p. 346): increased.

57  (a)  False (p. 364): it is a semistructured interview.
    (b)  True (p. 364).
    (c)  False (p. 364): it scores content and vocal tone.
    (d)  True (p. 364).
    (e)  False (p. 364): included.

58 The following are clinical features of tardive dyskinesia:

(a) The 'bon bon' sign.
(b) The 'flycatcher' sign.
(c) Bruxism.
(d) Trismus.
(e) Restless legs.

59 The following are true of akathisia:

(a) Movements are non-goal directed.
(b) It affects males and females approximately equally.
(c) Prevalence is approximately 25%.
(d) It often responds to anticholinergics.
(e) It refers to the inability to sit and stand still.

60 The following are true:

(a) Impairment refers to a restriction in functioning.
(b) Impairment results from handicap.
(c) Disability is a loss of psychological, physiological or anatomical structure or function.
(d) Handicap results from impairment or disability.
(e) Disability limits the fulfilment of a role that is normal for that individual.

61 Basic techniques of skills training in chronic schizophrenia include:

(a) Prompting.
(b) Modelling.
(c) Shaping.
(d) Positive reinforcement.
(e) Behavioural rehearsal.

62 Schizoaffective disorder:

(a) Affective symptoms must precede schizophrenic symptoms for ICD–10 criteria to be met.
(b) The course must be recurrent for ICD–10 criteria to be met.
(c) ICD–10 excludes patients with separate episodes of schizophrenia and affective disorder.
(d) Lithium prophylaxis is as effective for schizoaffective manic disorder as it is for mania.
(e) DSM–IV criteria include at least 2 weeks of delusions and hallucinations without prominent mood disorder.

58   (a)  True  (p. 437).
     (b)  True  (p. 437).
     (c)  True  (p. 437).
     (d)  True  (p. 437).
     (e)  True  (p. 437).

59   (a)  True  (p. 434).
     (b)  False  (p. 434): female:male ratio is 2:1.
     (c)  True  (p. 434): 21–32%.
     (d)  False  (p. 435).
     (e)  True  (p. 434): strictly incorrect – the term tasikinesia refers to the inability to sit still.

60   (a)  False (p. 458): loss or abnormality of psychological, physiological or anatomical structure or function.
     (b)  False (p. 458): handicap results from impairment.
     (c)  False (p. 458): this is the definition of an impairment.
     (d)  True (p. 458).
     (e)  False (p. 458): handicap limits the fulfilment of a role that is normal for that individual.

61   (a)  True  (p. 470).
     (b)  True  (p. 470).
     (c)  True  (p. 470).
     (d)  True  (p. 470).
     (e)  True  (p. 470).

62   (a)  False (p. 490): simultaneous presentation and both prominent.
     (b)  True  (p. 490).
     (c)  True  (p. 490).
     (d)  True  (p. 493).
     (e)  True  (p. 490).

63  The diagnostic guidelines for cycloid psychosis include:
(a)  Occurring for the first time in subjects aged 15–50 years.
(b)  Insidious deterioration over 1 month.
(c)  Mood-congruent delusions.
(d)  Motility disturbances.
(e)  A particular concern with death.

64  The following are delusions of misidentification:
(a)  Capgras syndrome.
(b)  Fregoli syndrome.
(c)  Subjective doubles syndrome.
(d)  Intermetamorphosis syndrome.
(e)  *Folie à deux*.

65  Suicide:
(a)  The profile of the incidence of suicide across all social classes forms a U-shaped curve.
(b)  Upper social classes have the highest suicide mortality.
(c)  The risk of suicide is greater in personality disorder than in schizophrenia.
(d)  Adverse life events are probably not especially common before suicide.
(e)  Higher rates of suicide are negatively correlated with unemployment.

66  Correlates of deliberate self-harm include:
(a)  Social class III.
(b)  Overcrowded accommodation.
(c)  At present address less than 1 year.
(d)  Males under 18 years.
(e)  Significant debts.

67  Risk factors for suicide in patients admitted to hospital following deliberate self-harm include:
(a)  Female gender.
(b)  Advancing age in men.
(c)  Long-term use of hypnotics.
(d)  Repeated attempts.
(e)  Absence of psychiatric disorder.

68  The following conditions are classified under anxiety disorders in ICD–10:
(a)  Social phobia.
(b)  Agoraphobia.
(c)  Post-traumatic stress disorder (PTSD).
(d)  Acute stress disorder.
(e)  Substance-induced anxiety disorder.

63   (a)   True   (p. 494).
     (b)   False   (p. 494): sudden onset.
     (c)   False   (p. 495): mood incongruent.
     (d)   True   (p. 495).
     (e)   True   (p. 495).

64   (a)   True   (p. 508).
     (b)   True   (p. 508).
     (c)   True   (p. 508).
     (d)   True   (p. 508).
     (e)   False   (p. 508).

65   (a)   True   (p. 520).
     (b)   True   (p. 520).
     (c)   False   (p. 518): the reverse is true – the risk of suicide is higher in schizophrenia than in personality disorder.
     (d)   False   (p. 520).
     (e)   False   (p. 520): positively correlated.

66   (a)   False   (p. 539): social class V.
     (b)   True   (p. 539).
     (c)   True   (p. 539).
     (d)   False   (p. 539): females under 23 years.
     (e)   True   (p. 539).

67   (a)   False   (p. 547).
     (b)   False   (p. 547): in women only.
     (c)   True   (p. 547).
     (d)   True   (p. 547).
     (e)   False   (p. 547): presence of psychiatric disorder.

68   (a)   False   (p. 558): phobic disorder, but DSM–IV does classify it as an anxiety disorder.
     (b)   False   (p. 558): phobic disorder.
     (c)   False   (p. 558): although this is correct for DSM–IV.
     (d)   False   (p. 558): although this is correct for DSM–IV.
     (e)   False   (p. 558): although this is correct for DSM–IV.

69  PTSD:

(a)  Intrusive memories tend to be of short duration and the subject remains in touch with reality.
(b)  The Impact of Events Scale has three sub-scales.
(c)  Acute stress reaction is similar to PTSD in terms of duration.
(d)  ICD–10 specifies that onset should be within 6 months of trauma.
(e)  Benzodiazepines have little effect on core PTSD symptoms.

70  Anxiety disorders have the following features:

(a)  The prevalence of panic disorder is the same in males and females aged over 30 years.
(b)  The Hamilton Anxiety Scale is observer rated.
(c)  Phobic disorder appears to be the most strongly genetically determined subtype of anxiety.
(d)  Panic is induced by sodium lactate infusion in 40% of patients with panic disorder or agoraphobia.
(e)  Propranolol blocks yohimbine-induced anxiety.

71  The features of agoraphobia:

(a)  Agoraphobia accounts for 60% of phobias.
(b)  At least two-thirds of patients are women.
(c)  Relatives of patients with agoraphobia have a raised risk of panic disorder and not other phobias.
(d)  Generalised anxiety is uncommon in agoraphobia.
(e)  Patients are usually aged 15–25 years.

72  The following are associated with obsessive–compulsive disorder (OCD):

(a)  Head injury.
(b)  Anorexia nervosa.
(c)  Schizophrenia.
(d)  Gilles de la Tourette syndrome.
(e)  Encephalitis lethargica.

73  In relation to OCD the following statements are true:

(a)  It has an equal gender ratio.
(b)  Women more commonly suffer from checking rituals.
(c)  Age of onset is earlier in women than in men.
(d)  Onset is usually in childhood.
(e)  Approximately 50% of all patients who present for treatment are unmarried.

69　(a)　True　(p. 568).
　　(b)　False (p. 570): two sub-scales – intrusion and avoidance. It has 15 items.
　　(c)　False (p. 570): acute stress reaction usually resolves within 4 weeks.
　　(d)　True　(p. 572).
　　(e)　True　(p. 576): reduce anxiety only.

70　(a)　True　(pp. 582–583).
　　(b)　False (p. 581): it is self-rated.
　　(c)　False (p. 584): panic.
　　(d)　False (p. 585): 75%.
　　(e)　False (p. 586): diazepam and clonidine block yohimbine-induced anxiety.

71　(a)　True　(p. 629).
　　(b)　True　(p. 629).
　　(c)　False (p. 629): raised for agoraphobia, panic disorder and other phobias.
　　(d)　False (p. 631).
　　(e)　False (p. 629): 15–35 years.

72　(a)　True　(p. 657).
　　(b)　True　(p. 656).
　　(c)　True　(p. 656).
　　(d)　True　(p. 656).
　　(e)　True　(p. 657).

73　(a)　True　(p. 658).
　　(b)　False (p. 658): compulsive washing and avoidance are commoner in women; checking rituals are commoner in men.
　　(c)　False (p. 658): age of onset is earlier in men than women.
　　(d)　False (p. 658): early adult life.
　　(e)　True　(p. 658).

74   Globus hystericus:

(a)   Is exacerbated by eating.
(b)   Is often associated with weight loss.
(c)   May be associated with dry swallowing.
(d)   Is, by definition, excluded by the presence of physiological anomalies.
(e)   Is often localised to the crico-pharyngeal level.


75   The features of Ganser syndrome include:

(a)   Memory defect.
(b)   Clear consciousness.
(c)   Perplexity.
(d)   Hallucinations.
(e)   Hysterical motor and sensory symptoms.


76   Hysterical blindness:

(a)   Hysterical blindness is common in ophthalmological practice.
(b)   It is often partial.
(c)   It is often associated with tubular or spiral visual fields.
(d)   Evoked potential studies are frequently abnormal.
(e)   Opto-kinetic nystagmus is more likely to occur than not.


77   Hypochondriacal disorder, as defined in ICD–10, has the following features:

(a)   Lack of response to medical reassurance.
(b)   Persistent preoccupation with physical appearance.
(c)   Adults with hypochondriasis often have had a model in childhood for their symptoms.
(d)   The Whiteley index is a measure of hysteria.
(e)   It is over-represented in social class V.


78   Dysmorphophobia:

(a)   The diagnostic criteria specify that it occurs in the absence of a physical anomaly.
(b)   May be a generalised disturbance of body image.
(c)   There may be a preoccupation with more than one body part at the same time.
(d)   Resistance to thought is common.
(e)   It is often a symptom of other psychiatric disorder, especially schizophrenia.


79   Munchhausen's syndrome by proxy:

(a)   The history presented suggests a multisystem disorder rather than a single-system disorder.
(b)   The father is the perpetrator in only 10% of cases.
(c)   Approximately 40% of these mothers had Munchhausen's syndrome.
(d)   Symptoms have usually persisted or recurred for periods of more than 1 year.
(e)   Children are exposed to iatrogenic harm.

74 (a) False (p. 687): it disappears with eating.
   (b) False (p. 687).
   (c) True (p. 687).
   (d) False (p. 687).
   (e) True (p. 687).

75 (a) True (p. 692).
   (b) False (p. 692): clouded consciousness.
   (c) True (p. 692).
   (d) True (p. 692).
   (e) True (p. 692).

76 (a) True (p. 689).
   (b) True (p. 689).
   (c) True (p. 689).
   (d) False (p. 689).
   (e) True (p. 689).

77 (a) True (p. 713).
   (b) True (p. 713).
   (c) True (p. 718).
   (d) False (p. 720): it is not a feature, but a measure of hysteria; see also Illness Attitude Test, Illness Behaviour Inventory.
   (e) False (p. 718): it occurs in all classes.

78 (a) False (p. 727): a slight anomaly may be present but the person's concern is markedly excessive.
   (b) False (p. 727).
   (c) True (p. 727).
   (d) True (p. 727): but not always present.
   (e) True (p. 727).

79 (a) True (p. 743).
   (b) False (p. 743): 5%.
   (c) False (p. 744): 20%.
   (d) True (p. 743).
   (e) True (p. 743).

80 The following are names of categories of personality disorder in ICD–10:
(a) Schizotypal.
(b) Antisocial.
(c) Narcissistic.
(d) Obsessive–compulsive.
(e) Avoidant.

81 ICD–10 criteria for anankastic personality disorder include:
(a) Tendency to bear grudges.
(b) Combative sense of personal rights.
(c) Excessively pedantic and adherent to social conventions.
(d) Feelings of doubt and caution.
(e) Intrusion of insistent unwelcome thoughts or impulses.

82 ICD–10 criteria for paranoid personality disorder include:
(a) Excessive social anxiety
(b) Recurrent suspicion of sexual partners, without justification.
(c) Excess self-importance and self-referential attitude.
(d) Lack of close friends or only one.
(e) Ideas of reference.

83 ICD–10 criteria for schizoid personality disorder include:
(a) Few if any activities provide pleasure.
(b) Limited capacity to express warmth.
(c) Little interest in sexual experience.
(d) Preoccupied with unsubstantiated conspiratorial explanations.
(e) Excessive social anxiety.

84 Epidemiological features of antisocial personality disorder:
(a) There is a lifetime prevalence of 3%.
(b) The male:female ratio is 1:1.
(c) Rates are independent of environment.
(d) Rates are independent of religious factors.
(e) An effect for lower social classes is significant.

85 ICD–10 criteria for dissocial personality disorder include:
(a) The individual must be at least 18 years of age.
(b) There should be evidence of conduct disorder before the age of 15 years.
(c) The antisocial behaviour should not occur exclusively in the course of schizophrenia or a manic episode.
(d) There should be difficulty in establishing relationships.
(e) There should be a marked proneness to offer plausible, rational explanations.

80  (a)  False (p. 759): schizotypal disorder is classified in the section on schizophrenia.
    (b)  False (p. 759): there is though 'dissocial' in ICD–10.
    (c)  False (p. 759).
    (d)  False (p. 759): there is though 'anankastic' in ICD–10.
    (e)  False (p. 759): there is though 'anxious' in ICD–10.
         Note. All of these are in DSM–IV.

81  (a)  False (p. 770): this is a feature of paranoid personality disorder.
    (b)  False (p. 770): this is a feature of paranoid personality disorder.
    (c)  True (p. 769).
    (d)  True (p. 769).
    (e)  True (p. 769).

82  (a)  False (p. 773): this is a feature of DSM–IV schizotypal personality disorder.
    (b)  True (p. 770).
    (c)  True (p. 770).
    (d)  False (p. 772): this is a feature of schizoid personality disorder.
    (e)  False (p. 773): this is a DSM–IV criterion for schizotypal personality disorder.

83  (a)  True (p. 772).
    (b)  True (p. 772).
    (c)  True (p. 772).
    (d)  False (p. 770): this is a feature of paranoid personality disorder.
    (e)  False (p. 773): this is a DSM–IV criterion for schizotypal personality disorder.

84  (a)  True (p. 774): 2–3%.
    (b)  False (p. 775): 6:1 to 2.6:1.
    (c)  False (p. 775): higher in urban than rural environments.
    (d)  False (p. 774): sociocultural and religious factors may influence the rate.
    (e)  False (p. 775): likely to be small.

85  (a)  False (p. 778): This is a DSM–IV criterion.
    (b)  False (p. 778): DSM–IV criterion.
    (c)  False (p. 778): DSM–IV criterion.
    (d)  False (p. 778): incapacity to maintain enduring relationships.
    (e)  True (p. 778): also to blame others.

86   Aetiology of antisocial personality disorder:
(a)   Twin and adoption studies all point to a significant hereditary contribution.
(b)   Electroencephalographic abnormalities include increased delta activity.
(c)   In a comparison between primary and secondary psychopaths, primary psychopaths have more rapid electrodermal habituation.
(d)   Higher levels of CSF 5-HIAA have been found in arsonists.
(e)   40% of children with a conduct disorder will later develop antisocial personality disorder.

87   ICD–10 criteria for histrionic personality disorder include:
(a)   Suggestibility.
(b)   Considering relationships to be more intimate than they actually are.
(c)   Excessively impressionistic speech style.
(d)   Overconcerned with physical attractiveness.
(e)   Exaggerated expression of emotion.

88   ICD–10 criteria for dependent personality disorder include:
(a)   Difficulty in initiating projects on his or her own.
(b)   Volunteers to do things that are unpleasant or demeaning to get others to like him or her.
(c)   Shallow and labile affectivity.
(d)   Identity disturbance.
(e)   Unwillingness to make even reasonable demands on others.

89   Assessment of personality disorder:
(a)   The Standardised Assessment of Personality is a self-report questionnaire.
(b)   The Personality Assessment Schedule generates ICD–10 diagnoses.
(c)   In the Personality Assessment Schedule interview emphasis is placed on the patient's premorbid traits.
(d)   The Eysenck Personality Inventory is a structured interview.
(e)   'Harria-parmia' is one of 16 dimensions in Cattell's 16PF.

90   Trichotillomania:
(a)   Is not uncommon, occurring in 1% of new psychiatric referrals.
(b)   Occurs in males and females equally.
(c)   May be exacerbated by substance misuse.
(d)   Is associated with personality disorder.
(e)   Is associated with an increased lifetime prevalence of major depression.

91   The following are ICD–10 criteria for anorexia nervosa:
(a)   Fear of fatness.
(b)   Failure of weight gain.
(c)   Excessive exercise.
(d)   Reduced $T_3$.
(e)   Avoidance of carbohydrate foods.

86  (a)  True  (p. 779).
    (b)  False  (p. 780): increased theta activity only partially replicated.
    (c)  False  (p. 780): true for secondary psychopaths, who also have lower cortical arousal and fewer spontaneous fluctuations on skin conductance.
    (d)  False  (p. 780): lower.
    (e)  True  (p. 781).

87  (a)  True  (p. 789).
    (b)  False  (p. 789): this is a DSM–IV criterion.
    (c)  False  (p. 789): DSM–IV criterion. Speech is also lacking in detail.
    (d)  True  (p. 789).
    (e)  True  (p. 789).

88  (a)  False  (p. 793): this is a DSM–IV criterion.
    (b)  False  (p. 793): DSM–IV criterion.
    (c)  False  (p. 789): ICD–10 criterion for histrionic personality disorder.
    (d)  False  (p. 784): DSM–IV criterion for borderline personality disorder.
    (e)  True  (p. 793).

89  (a)  False  (p. 799): relies on informant to provide description of the patient when well.
    (b)  True  (p. 799).
    (c)  True  (p. 799): it requires either the subject or informant or both to provide information on 24 traits of personality.
    (d)  False  (p. 799): it is self-rated, and comprises 108 questions related to dimensions of neuroticism, extroversion, psychoticism and a lie scale.
    (e)  True  (p. 799).

90  (a)  True  (p. 804).
    (b)  False  (p. 804): marked female predominance.
    (c)  True  (p. 804): also true of depression.
    (d)  False  (p. 804).
    (e)  True  (p. 804): also true of simple phobia, generalised anxiety disorder and possibly alcoholism and substance misuse.

91  (a)  True  (p. 863).
    (b)  True  (p. 863): or significant weight loss.
    (c)  True  (p. 863).
    (d)  True  (p. 863).
    (e)  False  (p. 863): avoidance of fattening foods.

92 The following are endocrine abnormalities in anorexia nervosa:
(a) The hypothalamic–pituitary–gonadal axis regresses to a pubertal state.
(b) Luteinising hormone (LH) but not follicle-stimulating hormone (FSH) is reduced.
(c) Oestrogen and progesterone levels are undetectable.
(d) Pelvic ultrasound reveals enlarged multi-follicular ovaries.
(e) Levels of magnesium are reduced.

93 Metabolic features of anorexia nervosa:
(a) Asymptomatic hypoglycaemia is often found.
(b) Raised cholesterol level may reflect the high-fat diet.
(c) Plasma potassium occasionally falls below 3 mmol/l.
(d) Sodium is invariably reduced.
(e) Intravenous potassium is likely to be required if potassium level is less than 2 mmol/l.

94 The following blood chemistry findings occur in anorexia nervosa:
(a) Raised or lowered urea.
(b) Raised or lowered bicarbonate.
(c) Salivary amylase isoenzyme increased.
(d) Raised or lowered phosphate.
(e) Lowered globulin.

95 The following blood hormone changes occur in anorexia nervosa:
(a) Decreased FSH and LH.
(b) Increased salivary amylase.
(c) Increased reverse $T_4$.
(d) Increased prolactin.
(e) Raised basal insulin.

96 Haematological manifestations of anorexia nervosa:
(a) Leucopenia is common.
(b) A haemoglobin of 9 g/100 ml due to marrow suppression is common.
(c) Thrombocytopenia is raised.
(d) The erythrocyte sedimentation rate (ESR) is raised.
(e) Carotene level is raised.

97 CNS findings of anorexia nervosa include:
(a) Capacity for complex thought remains intact, but concentration is impaired.
(b) Cerebral atrophy.
(c) Ventricular decrease.
(d) Widened sulci.
(e) Resolution of CNS structural changes in most cases following weight gain.

92   (a)   False (p. 868): pre-pubertal.
     (b)   False (p. 868): both.
     (c)   True (p. 868).
     (d)   False (p. 868): small multi-follicular ovaries and a small uterus.
     (e)   False (p. 871): sometimes decreased magnesium levels.

93   (a)   True (p. 868): does not require active management other than usual refeeding regime.
     (b)   False (p. 868, p. 871): may be caused by altered oestrogen and thyroid hormone metabolism – people with anorexia nervosa opt for a low-fat diet.
     (c)   True (p. 871).
     (d)   False (p. 871): is sometimes reduced, as are magnesium and phosphate.
     (e)   False (p. 871).

94   (a)   True (p. 870): low in restricting anorexia nervosa; raised with vomiting and laxative abuse.
     (b)   True (p. 870): raised to over 30 mmol/l with vomiting; less than 18 mmol/l occurs with laxative misuse.
     (c)   True (p. 870).
     (d)   False (p. 870): decreased phosphate only.
     (e)   True (p. 870): albumin and globulin may be lowered.

95   (a)   True (p. 870).
     (b)   False (p. 870): isoenzyme.
     (c)   False (p. 870): increased reverse $T_3$ and decreased $T_4$.
     (d)   False (p. 870): normal prolactin.
     (e)   False (p. 870): reduced basal insulin but increased sensitivity to insulin.

96   (a)   True (p. 871): white cell counts less than 4000 are common.
     (b)   True (p. 871).
     (c)   True (p. 870).
     (d)   False (p. 871): lowered ESR.
     (e)   False (p. 870): not a haematological finding (but true nevertheless).

97   (a)   False (p. 871): both impaired.
     (b)   True (p. 871).
     (c)   False (p. 871): dilatation.
     (d)   True (p. 871).
     (e)   True (p. 871).

98 Medical indications for admission of patients with anorexia nervosa include:
(a) Body mass index below 13.5 kg/m$^2$.
(b) Hypoglycaemia.
(c) Petechial rash and platelet suppression.
(d) Proximal myopathy.
(e) Risk of suicide.

99 ICD–10 criteria for bulimia nervosa include:
(a) A minimum of 2 binges per week over 3 months.
(b) Morbid fear of fatness with a sharply defined weight threshold.
(c) Episodes of overeating.
(d) A link with anorexia nervosa although not essential for diagnosis.
(e) Feeling of lack of control of eating during binge.

100 The following are true of bulimia nervosa:
(a) The median age of onset is 18 years.
(b) Approximately one-third of patients have a history of obesity.
(c) Patients are frequently of normal body weight.
(d) The gender ratio is similar to that in anorexia nervosa.
(e) Bulimia is over-represented among ballet dancers, models and actresses.

101 The following occur in bulimia nervosa:
(a) Self-mutilation in 25%.
(b) Suicide attempts in 10%.
(c) Promiscuity in 20%.
(d) Shoplifting in 20%.
(e) Alcohol misuse in 10%.

102 The following statements are true regarding bulimia nervosa:
(a) The BITE is a widely used self- and observer-report questionnaire.
(b) Approximately 25% of alcoholic patients have a history of an eating disorder.
(c) Bulimia nervosa is five to ten times commoner than anorexia nervosa.
(d) The combination of vomiting and laxative abuse can lead to the unusual combination of hypokalaemia and alkalosis.
(e) There is a recovery rate of 50–70% after 2–5 years of illness.

103 Puerperal psychosis:
(a) In most cases there is a symptom-free latent interval during the first 2 or 3 days.
(b) Puerperal psychosis may be associated with a mild fever commonly associated with infection.
(c) The onset is generally abrupt.
(d) Sleep is invariably severely disturbed in puerperal mania.
(e) Approximately 50% of women admitted for puerperal psychosis are suffering from a depressive disorder.

98 (a) True (p. 879): or a rapid rate of fall.
   (b) True (p. 879): symptomatic hypoglycaemia.
   (c) True (p. 879).
   (d) True (p. 879).
   (e) False (p. 879): psychiatric indication.

99 (a) False (p. 885): this is a DSM–IV criterion – frequency criteria are not present in ICD–10.
   (b) True (p. 886).
   (c) True (p. 886).
   (d) True (p. 885).
   (e) True (p. 885).

100 (a) True (p. 885).
   (b) True (p. 885): also one-third have a history of anorexia nervosa.
   (c) True (p. 885).
   (d) True (p. 885).
   (e) True (p. 885).

101 (a) False (p. 887): 10%.
   (b) False (p. 887): 30%.
   (c) False (p. 887): 10%.
   (d) True (p. 887).
   (e) True (p. 887): 10–15%.

102 (a) False (p. 887): self-report only.
   (b) False (pp. 887, 888): approximately one-third to one-half.
   (c) True (p. 888).
   (d) False (p. 889): hypokalaemia and acidosis.
   (e) True (p. 895).

103 (a) False (p. 904): in some cases only – it commonly starts on the fourth or fifth day.
   (b) False (p. 904): rarely associated with infection.
   (c) False (p. 905): may be abrupt but more often there is increasing irritability or elation.
   (d) True (p. 905).
   (e) True (p. 905).

104 The following drugs are safe to give to a breastfeeding mother:

(a) Trazodone.
(b) Doxepin.
(c) Fluoxetine.
(d) Zopiclone.
(e) Phenytoin.

105 Maternity blues:

(a) Maternity blues occur in 40–50% of mothers.
(b) 10% of sufferers report hypnopompic hallucinations.
(c) REM sleep may show a rebound increase on nights 2–3 post-partum.
(d) The blues generally last 3 days.
(e) Previous premenstrual tension is an established clinical association.

106 Hormonal and biochemical hypothesis of maternity blues:

(a) Maternity blues may be explained by the relative sharp rise in progesterone following delivery.
(b) The sharp drop in oestrogen levels fails to correlate with mood disturbance.
(c) An association between the blues and reduced plasma cortisol levels has been reported.
(d) During the early puerperium over 80% of women are dexamethasone suppressors.
(e) Body weight continues to rise for the first 3 days post-partum.

107 Edinburgh Postnatal Depression Scale:

(a) Consists of 20 items.
(b) Can be administered by health visitors.
(c) Consists of a mood adjective checklist.
(d) Is a self-rating scale.
(e) Comprises mainly neurotic symptoms.

108 The following symptoms occur at a frequency of at least 20% in premenstrual syndrome:

(a) Bloatedness.
(b) Anxiety and panic.
(c) Skin lesions.
(d) Alcohol craving.
(e) Urinary symptoms.

109 The following statements are true regarding delirium:

(a) Onset is often insidious.
(b) It is worse at night.
(c) Level of alertness is usually abnormally low or high.
(d) Primary or working memory is shortened.
(e) Autonomic changes are unusual.

104 (a) True (p. 914).
   (b) False (p. 914): accumulation of doxepin metabolite may cause sedation.
   (c) True (p. 914): only small amounts in breast milk but it may accumulate in the infant, although this is now not regarded as important.
   (d) False (p. 914): excreted in appreciable amounts in breast milk.
   (e) True (p. 915): carbamazepine is also safe; valproate should be used with caution at high doses.

105 (a) False (p. 929): 50–70%.
   (b) True (p. 929).
   (c) True (p. 929): REM and stage 4 sleep are decreased in pregnancy.
   (d) False (p. 930): brief acute episode lasting for no more than a few hours for 1 or 2 days only.
   (e) True (p. 930): maternity blues are also associated with anxiety and depression during late pregnancy and subsequent postnatal depression.

106 (a) False (p. 930): sharp drop occurs.
   (b) True (p. 931).
   (c) False (p. 931): elevated plasma cortisol.
   (d) False (p. 931): non-suppressors.
   (e) True (p. 931): and then abruptly falls on day 4.

107 (a) False (p. 932): 13 items.
   (b) True (p. 932).
   (c) False (p. 932): Kennerly and Gath scale consists of a mood adjective checklist.
   (d) True (p. 932).
   (e) True (p. 932): Stein also described a 13-item scale comprising mainly neurotic symptoms.

108 (a) True (p. 941).
   (b) False (p. 941).
   (c) False (p. 941).
   (d) False (p. 941).
   (e) False (p. 941).

   Note. Depression, irritability, tiredness, headaches and breast tenderness are among the commoner symptoms.

109 (a) False (p. 960): acute; dementia is usually insidious.
   (b) True (p. 960).
   (c) True (p. 960).
   (d) True (p. 960).
   (e) False (p. 960): they are common.

110 The following are true of dementia:

(a) Dementia is characterised by a fluctuating course.
(b) Attention is often impaired.
(c) Anomia is common.
(d) Autonomic changes are unusual.
(e) The electroencephalogram shows diffuse slow-wave activity.

111 The features of frontal lobe syndrome include:

(a) Preservation of IQ.
(b) Moria.
(c) Preservation of judgement of temporal order.
(d) Contralateral optic atrophy.
(e) Preservation of the ability to shift cognitive set.

112 Temporal lobe syndrome:

(a) A lesion of the non-dominant temporal lobe may produce Wernicke's aphasia alone.
(b) Bilateral medial temporal lobe lesions produce a severe and selective amnesic syndrome.
(c) More posterior lesions tend to produce alexia and agraphia.
(d) There is support for an association of schizophrenia-like psychosis and right-sided epileptic foci.
(e) The single most important sign of a deep temporal lobe lesion is a contralateral lower quadrantic hemianopia.

113 Kluver–Bucy syndrome has the following features:

(a) Follows bilateral ablation of lateral temporal lobes.
(b) Excessive oral tendencies including bulimia.
(c) Aggressiveness.
(d) Prosopagnosia.
(e) Hypometamorphosis.

114 Parietal lobe syndromes:

(a) Lesions of the non-dominant lobe produce conduction aphasia.
(b) Posterior dominant lesions may be associated with motor dysphasia.
(c) Anterior dominant lesions may be associated with sensory dysphasia.
(d) Dominant parietal lobe lesions produce disturbances of body image.
(e) Anterior lesions cause contralateral cortical sensory loss.

115 Features of occipital lobe lesions include:

(a) Characteristic contralateral homonymous defects.
(b) Characteristic complex visual recognition disorders.
(c) Colour agnosia.
(d) Alexia and agraphia.
(e) Elementary visual hallucinations.

110 (a) False (p. 960): stable over days.
   (b) False (p. 960): relatively normal.
   (c) True (p. 960).
   (d) True (p. 960).
   (e) False (p. 960): diffuse slow-wave activity is present in delirium. Mild slowing can occur in dementia but it varies with the aetiology.

111 (a) True (p. 964): also true for memory and other cognitive functions.
   (b) True (p. 964): 'moria' is silliness, also puns and pranks.
   (c) False (p. 965): impaired.
   (d) False (p. 965): ipsilateral – also focal seizures, anosmia, grasp reflex and Broca's aphasia.
   (e) False (p. 965): loss, as revealed by Wisconsin Card-Sorting Test.

112 (a) False (p. 965): this occurs with dominant temporal lobe lesions.
   (b) True (p. 965).
   (c) True (p. 965).
   (d) False (p. 965): left-sided epileptic foci.
   (e) False (p. 966): upper quadrantic.

113 (a) False (p. 966): Kluver–Bucy syndrome follows ablation of the medial and lateral temporal lobes, including amygdalae unci and hippocampi. It also follows lesions.
   (b) True (p. 966).
   (c) False (p. 966): it includes placidity and pet-like compliance.
   (d) True (p. 966): it includes prosopagnosia (sometimes) and visual agnosia.
   (e) False (p. 966): it includes hypermetamorphosis, which is an irresistible impulse to touch objects.

114 (a) False (p. 968): dominant lobe.
   (b) False (p. 968): sensory dysphasia.
   (c) False (p. 968): motor dysphasia.
   (d) False (p. 968).
   (e) True (p. 968).

115 (a) True (p. 968).
   (b) False (p. 968): less common.
   (c) True (p. 968).
   (d) False (p. 968): alexia without agraphia.
   (e) False (p. 968): complex.

116 Lesions of deep midline structures (diencephalon and brain-stem) include:
(a) Characteristic amnesic syndrome.
(b) Characteristic hypersomnia.
(c) Hydrocephalus.
(d) Frontal-type syndrome.
(e) Characteristic focal neurological signs.

117 Aphasia:
(a) Left-hemisphere dominance for language occurs in 90% of right-handed people.
(b) Patients with disturbed repetition have perisylvian pathology.
(c) Non-fluent aphasia is associated with pathology posterior to the major central sulcus.
(d) Fluent aphasia indicates pathology in Wernicke's area.
(e) The hallmark of conduction aphasia is impairment of repetition of speech out of proportion to all other deficits.

118 Features of primary motor aphasia include:
(a) Fluent paraphasic speech.
(b) Grimacing and gestures.
(c) Dysprosody.
(d) Logorrhoea.
(e) Perseveration.

119 Features of Wernicke's aphasia:
(a) Defective repetition.
(b) Patient speaks effortlessly and without hesitation.
(c) Normal prosody.
(d) Phonemic paraphasias are a major type of error.
(e) Naming ability is usually poor and, in contrast to motor aphasia, prompting rarely helps.

120 Anomic aphasia:
(a) Confrontation naming is affected more than any other language function.
(b) Low-frequency names are particularly affected.
(c) It is an early symptom in dementia.
(d) It raises the possibility of a lesion in the left hemisphere.
(e) It occurs occasionally in hysteria.

116 (a) True (p. 969).
    (b) True (p. 969).
    (c) True (p. 969): leading to generalised intellectual decline.
    (d) True (p. 969).
    (e) False (p. 969): may be absent.

117 (a) False (p. 969): this occurs in 95–99% of right-handed and 60–70% of left-handed people.
    (b) True (p. 969): that is, pathology in the primary language cortex; repetition is spared by surrounding cortical lesions.
    (c) False (p. 969): anterior to the major central sulcus.
    (d) True (p. 969).
    (e) True (p. 970).

118 (a) False (p. 970): spontaneous speech is non-fluent.
    (b) True (p. 970): demand increased effort to produce words.
    (c) True (p. 970): disturbance of rhythm.
    (d) False (p. 970): excessive speech is a feature of Wernicke's (or primary sensory) aphasia.
    (e) True (p. 970).

119 (a) True (p. 970): fluent paraphasic speech with defective repetition.
    (b) True (p. 970).
    (c) True (p. 970): rhythm, articulation and phrase length are normal.
    (d) True (p. 970): these are substitutions within language.
    (e) True (p. 970).

120 (a) True (p. 971).
    (b) True (p. 971): or words.
    (c) True (p. 971).
    (d) True (p. 971).
    (e) True (p. 971).

121 Alexia and agraphia:

(a) Alexia with agraphia implies both letter and numerical blindness plus word blindness.
(b) Spelling is intact in alexia without agraphia.
(c) The hallmark of alexia without agraphia is the inability of patients to read the words that they have just written.
(d) Associated findings include right homonymous hemianopia.
(e) The pathology involves the left occipital region.

122 Acquired reading disorders:

(a) Letter-by-letter dyslexia is accompanied by pronounced slowness in reading.
(b) Surface dyslexia is characterised by a particular difficulty in reading regular words.
(c) Surface dyslexia often results from left temporal lobe lesions.
(d) Deep dyslexia results from a defect of grapheme–phoneme conversion.
(e) Deep dyslexia is diagnosed by a particular difficulty in reading non-words.

123 Agnosia is a disorder of recognition of objects that cannot be attributed to the following:

(a) Sensory defects.
(b) Mental deterioration.
(c) Attentional disturbances.
(d) Aphasic misnaming.
(e) Unfamiliarity with the object.

124 Speech dominance and handedness:

(a) 5% of right-handers are right-hemisphere dominant.
(b) 15% of right-handers show a bilateral pattern of speech representation.
(c) Right-handers may have a better prognosis following cerebral vascular accidents involving language processes.
(d) The Annett Handedness Questionnaire is a commonly employed assessment of hand preference.
(e) There may be a higher prevalence of psychosis in mixed-handers and left-handers.

125 Features of the Gerstmann syndrome include:

(a) Non-dominant parietal lobe lesions.
(b) Bilateral loss of ability to recognise individual fingers.
(c) The patient cannot carry out instructions which involve an appreciation of right and left.
(d) The patient is unable to do simple additions.
(e) Dysaesthesia.

121 (a) True  (p. 971): all aspects of writing are affected.
    (b) True  (p. 971).
    (c) True  (p. 971).
    (d) True  (p. 971).
    (e) True  (p. 971): left inferior medial occipital region and splenium of corpus callosum.

122 (a) True  (p. 971): probably results from a visual processing deficit.
    (b) False  (pp. 971–972): irregular words.
    (c) True  (p. 972): for example in herpes encephalitis.
    (d) True  (p. 972).
    (e) True  (p. 972).

123 (a) True  (p. 973).
    (b) True  (p. 973).
    (c) True  (p. 973).
    (d) True  (p. 973).
    (e) True  (p. 973).

124 (a) True  (p. 974).
    (b) False  (p. 974): 15% of left-handers show a bilateral pattern of speech representation.
    (c) False  (p. 974): left-handers may have a better prognosis following cerebral vascular accidents involving language processes.
    (d) True  (p. 974).
    (e) True  (p. 974).

125 (a) False  (p. 975): dominant parietal lobe lesions.
    (b) True  (p. 975).
    (c) True  (p. 975).
    (d) True  (p. 975).
    (e) False  (p. 975): dysgraphia, dyscalculia, finger agnosia and right–left disorientation.

126 Body image disturbances:

(a) Bilateral body image disturbances are commoner with right cerebral lesions than left.
(b) Autopagnosia is a rare feature of bilateral body image disturbances.
(c) Unilateral body image disturbances more often affect the left side of the body.
(d) Anosognosia is much commoner for right-hemiplegic limbs.
(e) Unilateral unawareness is due to right parietal lobe lesions.

127 Visuospatial deficits:

(a) Bilateral occipitoparietal lesions result in visual disorientation.
(b) Visuospatial agnosia includes errors like misalignment of words on a page.
(c) Visuospatial agnosia is more common and severe with lesions of the left parietal lobe.
(d) Loss of topographical memory impairs the ability to recall or recognise routes, buildings or places.
(e) Difficulties occur with tactile maps.

128 Delirium:

(a) Disturbance of the sleep–wake cycle is an ICD–10 requirement for delirium.
(b) Loss of topographical memory is often seen.
(c) Thought processes are either slowed or rapid.
(d) Nominal dysphasia is common.
(e) Psychomotor activity is virtually always disturbed.

129 Lewy bodies are:

(a) Hyaline bodies.
(b) Eosinophilic.
(c) Intraneuronal inclusion bodies.
(d) Characteristically found in the substantia nigra of patients with Parkinson's disease.
(e) Found in the cerebral cortex of patients with dementia.

130 Features of Huntington's disease include:

(a) Cortical dementia.
(b) Insidious onset between 25 and 30 years of age.
(c) Juvenile form accounts for 10%.
(d) Interval between onset and diagnosis is approximately 5 years.
(e) Late-onset cases commonly present with mental changes.

126 (a) False (p. 975): commoner with left rather than right.
    (b) True (p. 975).
    (c) True (p. 975): commoner with right-hemisphere lesions.
    (d) False (p. 975): the term means lack of awareness of disease; it is much commoner for left-hemiplegic limbs.
    (e) True (p. 975).

127 (a) True (p. 976).
    (b) True (p. 976).
    (c) False (p. 976): commoner with the right parietal lobe.
    (d) True (p. 976).
    (e) True (p. 976): but not for all visual spatial deficits; also true for visual maps.

128 (a) True (p. 994).
    (b) True (p. 996).
    (c) True (p. 996).
    (d) True (p. 996).
    (e) True (p. 996).

129 (a) True (p. 1008).
    (b) True (p. 1008).
    (c) True (p. 1008).
    (d) True (p. 1008).
    (e) True (p. 1008).

130 (a) False (p. 1009): sub-cortical dementia.
    (b) False (p. 1010): between 35 and 45 years.
    (c) False (p. 1010): juvenile form accounts for 4%.
    (d) False (p. 1010): approximately 8 years.
    (e) False (p. 1010): chorea and few other features of Huntington's disease.

131 The following are correct in relation to Huntington's disease:
(a) Apraxia and agnosia are notably absent.
(b) The length of the responsible trinucleotide repeat and the age of onset are inversely correlated.
(c) Affected children have an age of onset 8–10 years earlier than their affected fathers.
(d) Patients with disease of paternal origin have more triplet repeats in the gene than those whose disease has been maternally transmitted.
(e) Affected children have an age of onset similar to that of their affected mothers.

132 Huntington's pathology includes:
(a) Caudate atrophy evident on computed tomography (CT).
(b) Spiny cell proliferation.
(c) Astrocytic depletion.
(d) Ventricular dilatation maximally affecting frontal area.
(e) Reduced levels of gamma-aminobutyric acid (GABA) in the striatal projection pathways in the frontal cortex.

133 In Huntington's disease the following transmitters are decreased:
(a) GABA in the basal ganglia.
(b) Met-enkephalin.
(c) Substance P.
(d) Cholecystokinin.
(e) Choline acetyltransferase.

134 In Creutzfeld–Jakob disease:
(a) Men and women are affected equally.
(b) The CSF is usually normal.
(c) 20% of cases have an autosomal dominant inheritance.
(d) Electroencephalography shows characteristic biphasic sharp-wave complexes.
(e) Myoclonic jerks occasionally occur.

135 In communicating hydrocephalus:
(a) The block is not within the ventricular system.
(b) Patients present with acute progressive dementia.
(c) Signs of raised intracranial pressure are absent.
(d) A history of headache is usual.
(e) It responds to ventricular drainage.

136 Epilepsy:
(a) Approximately 75% of focal seizures originate in the frontal area.
(b) An aura is a focal seizure.
(c) In adults the usual form of generalisation is a tonic–clonic seizure.
(d) In children 'absences' is the typical form of generalised seizures.
(e) Petit mal rarely starts after the age of 10 years.

131 (a) True (p. 1011).
 (b) True (p. 1011): regardless of the gender of the transmitting parent.
 (c) True (p. 1011).
 (d) True (p. 1011).
 (e) True (p. 1011).

132 (a) True (p. 1012): also progressive atrophy of the putamen.
 (b) False (p. 1012): spiny cell loss.
 (c) False (p. 1012): astrocytic proliferation.
 (d) True (p. 1012): also ventricular atrophy.
 (e) False (p. 1012): there are reduced levels of GABA in the basal ganglia and substantia nigra.

133 (a) True (p. 1012).
 (b) True (p. 1012).
 (c) True (p. 1012).
 (d) True (p. 1012).
 (e) True (p. 1012).

134 (a) True (p. 1013).
 (b) True (p. 1013).
 (c) False (p. 1013): 5–15%.
 (d) False (p. 1013): triphasic sharp-wave complexes.
 (e) False (p. 1013): they occur frequently.

135 (a) True (p. 1015): it is in the subarachnoid space, usually around the basal cisterns.
 (b) False (p. 1015): they present with subacute progressive dementia.
 (c) False (p. 1015): signs of raised intracranial pressure may be absent.
 (d) True (p. 1015): also ataxia and gait disturbance.
 (e) False (p. 1015): normal-pressure hydrocephalus may respond to ventricular drainage.

136 (a) False (p. 1032): approximately 75% of focal seizures originate in the temporal lobe, 15–20% in the frontal lobes, 5% in the parietal lobes and 3% in the occipital lobes.
 (b) True (p. 1030).
 (c) True (p. 1031).
 (d) True (p. 1031).
 (e) False (p. 1031): rarely after 20 years of age.

137 Epileptic aura:
(a) Visual illusions are typical in seizures of mesial temporal lobe origin.
(b) Oro-alimentary automatisms are characteristic of frontal lobe seizures.
(c) Scotomata suggest a seizure of parietal lobe origin.
(d) Speech arrest occurs in temporal lobe seizures.
(e) Sensory auras occur in parietal lobe seizures.

138 Features more often found in non-epileptic seizures include:
(a) A history of sexual maladjustment.
(b) The presence of a current affective disorder.
(c) Pelvic thrusting is particularly characteristic.
(d) Tongue-biting can occur.
(e) Non-stereotyped attack pattern.

139 Post-traumatic amnesia (PTA):
(a) PTA is the time from injury to restoration of memory, excluding islands of memory.
(b) A PTA of between 1 and 24 hours is regarded as severe.
(c) The length of PTA correlates well with eventual outcome.
(d) A PTA of less than 1 hour predicts return to work within 1 month.
(e) The PTA includes the length of period of confusion.

140 Cerebrovascular disease:
(a) Occlusion of the non-dominant middle cerebral artery may cause confusional states with few focal signs.
(b) Occlusion of the anterior cerebral artery causes denial of the disability.
(c) Occlusion of the post-cerebral artery causes cortical blindness.
(d) Occlusion of the rostral basilar artery can result in bizarre hallucinations.
(e) Occlusion of the post-cerebral artery causes alexia with agraphia.

141 Features of Friedreich's ataxia include:
(a) Autosomal dominant inheritance.
(b) Pes cavus.
(c) Hypertonicity.
(d) Personality changes.
(e) Cognitive impairment as a key presenting picture.

142 Feaures of dystrophia myotonica include:
(a) X-linked recessive inheritance.
(b) Pseudo-hypertrophy of lower leg.
(c) Typical abnormalities on electromyelography (EMG).
(d) Hypogonadism.
(e) 'Anticipation' in the genetic sense.

137 (a) False (p. 1032): visual illusions are typical in seizures of lateral temporal lobe origin.
   (b) False (p. 1032): oro-alimentary automatisms are characteristic of mesial temporal lobe seizures.
   (c) False (p. 1032): scotomata suggest an occipital lobe seizure.
   (d) False (p. 1032): speech arrest occurs in frontal lobe seizures.
   (e) True (p. 1032).

138 (a) True (p. 1042).
   (b) True (p. 1042).
   (c) True (p. 1042).
   (d) True (p. 1042).
   (e) True (p. 1042).

139 (a) True (p. 1047).
   (b) False (p. 1047): a PTA of between 1 and 24 hours is moderate, whereas a PTA greater than 24 hours is severe.
   (c) False (p. 1047): PTA length correlates very roughly with eventual outcome.
   (d) True (p. 1047).
   (e) True (p. 1047): also includes coma.

140 (a) True (p. 1054).
   (b) False (p. 1054): it may result in global dementia and frontal lobe personality changes.
   (c) True (p. 1054).
   (d) True (p. 1054): also disorientation and somnolence.
   (e) False (p. 1054): alexia without agraphia.

141 (a) False (p. 1060): autosomal recessive.
   (b) True (p. 1060).
   (c) False (p. 1060): hypotonicity.
   (d) True (p. 1060): especially immaturity and asociality.
   (e) False (p. 1060): no initial cognitive impairment.

142 (a) False (p. 1060): autosomal dominant. Duchenne muscular dystrophy is X-linked recessive.
   (b) False (p. 1060): pseudo-hypertrophy of lower leg is a feature of Duchenne's muscular dystrophy.
   (c) True (p. 1060).
   (d) True (p. 1060).
   (e) True (p. 1060): anticipation is worsening of the disorder over successive generations.

   Note. Other features include cataracts, cardiomyopathy, frontal balding and endocrine abnormalities.

143 Infection with the human immunodeficiency virus (HIV):
(a) Cerebral pathology is found in 90% of patients dying of AIDS.
(b) HIV-associated dementia occurs late in the course of infection in approximately 30% of patients.
(c) In AIDS dementia complex the electroencephalogram (EEG) has diffuse slowing.
(d) Neurophysiological evoked responses may demonstrate impaired subcortical function.
(e) Cortical focal deficits occur early.

144 Gilles de la Tourette syndrome:
(a) The syndrome is characterised by both multiple motor and one or more phonic tics.
(b) It usually begins before the age of 11 years.
(c) It occurs up to ten times more often in males than females.
(d) Coprolalia occurs in approximately one-third of sufferers.
(e) Palilalia occurs in approximately 10%.

145 Psychopathology of Gilles de la Tourette syndrome:
(a) The psychopathology most commonly recognised as characteristic of the condition is anxiety.
(b) The association with attention deficit disorder is as high as 90%.
(c) Self-injurious behaviour occurs in 10%.
(d) A verbal performance discrepancy of around 15 points is often found.
(e) Compulsions are more frequent than obsessions.

146 Investigations for Gilles de la Tourette syndrome:
(a) The principal abnormality in the EEG is the absence of the 'Bereitschafts' potential before the tics.
(b) Specific abnormalities in the visual and sensory evoked potentials have been found.
(c) Magnetic resonance imaging studies reveal abnormalities in the basal ganglia.
(d) Single-photon emission computed tomography shows hyperperfusion in the thalamic region.
(e) Paroxysmal activity synchronises with the tics on EMG.

147 Features of Wilson's disease include:
(a) Autosomal dominant inheritance.
(b) The responsible gene is on the long arm of chromosome 13.
(c) Most cases present in the first two decades.
(d) Rigidity is a common early sign.
(e) Tremor may be intention type or pill-rolling.

143 (a) True (p. 1069).
   (b) True (p. 1069).
   (c) True (p. 1069).
   (d) True (p. 1069).
   (e) False (p. 1069): they may be seen but are less common at first.

144 (a) True (p. 1078).
   (b) False (p. 1078): It usually begins before 18 years – and the mean age of onset is 11 years (p.1079).
   (c) False (p. 1078): 1.5–3 times more common in males.
   (d) False (p. 1079): occurs in less than 10% of people with Tourette syndrome.
   (e) True (p. 1079): 6–15%.

145 (a) False (p. 1080): obsessionality.
   (b) True (p. 1080): 20–90%.
   (c) False (p. 1080): one-third.
   (d) True (p. 1080).
   (e) True (p. 1080).

146 (a) False (p. 1082): true for EMG.
   (b) True (p. 1082).
   (c) True (p. 1082): also true for lateral ventricles.
   (d) False (p. 1082): hypoperfusion, also in the basal ganglia and frontal and temporal cortical areas.
   (e) False (p. 1082): EEG is essentially normal.

147 (a) False (p. 1083): autosomal recessive.
   (b) True (p. 1084).
   (c) True (p. 1084).
   (d) True (p. 1084): as is tremor.
   (e) True (p. 1085): most commonly it is a bizarre tremor described as 'wing beating'.

148 Investigations for Wilson's disease:

(a) Caeruloplasmin levels are high.
(b) Serum copper is usually low or normal.
(c) Urinary copper excretion is reduced.
(d) Magnetic resonance imaging shows ventricular dilatation.
(e) Slit-lamp examination is the definitive test for Kayser–Fleischer rings.

149 Risk factors for depression in Parkinson's disease include:

(a) Male gender.
(b) A family history of depression.
(c) Bradykinesis.
(d) Gait instability.
(e) A greater degree of right-brain involvement.

150 Psychiatric complications of levo-dopa include:

(a) Hyposexuality.
(b) Impulsivity.
(c) Vivid dreams.
(d) Anxiety.
(e) Agitation.

151 The main features of pathological alcohol intoxication include:

(a) Occurrence following the consumption of an unexpectedly small quantity of alcohol.
(b) Occurrence of irrational violence without psychosis.
(c) Occurrence of irrational violence without delirium.
(d) Occurrence of terminal sleep.
(e) Occurrence of a degree of amnesia for the events.

152 Hallucinations in alcohol states:

(a) Withdrawal hallucinations are usually associated with impaired cognition.
(b) Alcohol withdrawal hallucinations usually occur 12–48 hours into withdrawal.
(c) Characteristically they are most pronounced on the second night of withdrawal.
(d) They usually last for up to 1 hour.
(e) Insight is present.

153 Perceptual modality features in alcoholic hallucinations:

(a) Auditory features are the most prominent.
(b) Mixed auditory and visual occur in approximately 50% of cases.
(c) Alcohol withdrawal hallucinations infrequently become chronic.
(d) Third-person auditory hallucinations occur.
(e) In ICD–10 the disorder is classified in the alcohol section as a psychotic disorder.

148 (a)  False (p. 1086): low.
  (b)  True (p. 1086).
  (c)  False (p. 1086): generally elevated.
  (d)  True (p. 1086): also cortical atrophy and basal ganglia hypodensities.
  (e)  True (p. 1086).

149 (a)  False (p. 1089): female.
  (b)  False (p. 1089): personal history but not family history.
  (c)  True (p. 1089).
  (d)  True (pp. 1089–1090).
  (e)  False (p. 1090): left-brain involvement is more of a risk factor.

150 (a)  False (p. 1090): hypersexuality.
  (b)  True (p. 1090).
  (c)  True (p. 1090).
  (d)  True (p. 1090).
  (e)  True (p. 1090).

  Note. Complications also include psychosis, delirium, depression, lethargy and insomnia.

151 (a)  False (p. 1107): follows consumption of alcohol, possibly in an unexpectedly small quantity.
  (b)  False (p. 1107): with or without psychosis.
  (c)  False (p. 1107): with or without delirium.
  (d)  True (p. 1107).
  (e)  True (p. 1107).

152 (a)  False (p. 1110): not usually.
  (b)  True (p. 1110).
  (c)  False (p. 1110): first night.
  (d)  False (p. 1110): fleeting but may last several minutes.
  (e)  False (p. 1110): insight is variable.

153 (a)  False (p. 1111): visual features are the most prominent.
  (b)  False (p. 1111): approximately 26% of cases.
  (c)  True (p. 1111): in a minority.
  (d)  True (p. 1111).
  (e)  True (p. 1111): either as schizophrenia-like or predominantly hallucinatory.

154 Features of Wernicke's disease include:
(a) Bilateral medial rectus palsy.
(b) Divergent gaze palsy.
(c) Horizontal and/or vertical nystagmus.
(d) Impaired memory.
(e) A poly-neuropathy in which the legs alone are affected in most cases.

155 The features of Korsakoff's syndrome include:
(a) Preserved primary memory.
(b) Extensive retrograde amnesia.
(c) Absence of global cognitive impairment.
(d) Confabulation as a prerequisite for the diagnosis.
(e) Mild gait ataxia.

156 Symptoms of anticholinergic intoxication include:
(a) Sweating.
(b) Rhinorrhoea.
(c) Bradycardia.
(d) Reduced bowel sounds due to inhibition of parasympathetic control.
(e) Impairment of recent memory.

157 Features which are common to both anticholinergic intoxication and neuroleptic malignant syndrome are:
(a) Tachycardia.
(b) Dilated pupils.
(c) Dry skin.
(d) Hyperpyrexia.
(e) Labile blood pressure.

158 Clinical features of caffeine intoxication include:
(a) Rambling flow of thought and speech.
(b) Diuresis.
(c) Pallor.
(d) Headache.
(e) Hypersomnia.

159 Anorexia nervosa and hypopituitarism share the following:
(a) Significant weight loss.
(b) Impaired appetite.
(c) Amenorrhoea.
(d) Facial lanugo.
(e) Patient's attitude to food.

154 (a) False (p. 1115): lateral rectus.
   (b) False (p. 1115): conjugate gaze palsy.
   (c) True (p. 1115).
   (d) True (p. 1115).
   (e) True (p. 1115).

155 (a) True (p. 1115).
   (b) True (p. 1115).
   (c) True (p. 1115).
   (d) False (p. 1115): not a prerequisite.
   (e) False (p. 1115): this is a feature of Wernicke's disease.

156 (a) False (p. 1125): inhibition of sweating.
   (b) False (p. 1125): dry mouth.
   (c) False (p. 1125): tachycardia.
   (d) True (p. 1125).
   (e) True (p. 1126).

157 (a) True (p. 1126).
   (b) False (p. 1126): only anticholinergic intoxication.
   (c) False (p. 1126): only anticholinergic intoxication.
   (d) True (p. 1126).
   (e) True (p. 1126).

158 (a) True (p. 1131).
   (b) True (p. 1131).
   (c) False (p. 1131): flushed face.
   (d) False (p. 1131): withdrawal symptom.
   (e) False (p. 1131): withdrawal symptom.

159 (a) False (p. 1151): weight loss is usually less in hypopituitarism.
   (b) True (p. 1151).
   (c) True (p. 1151).
   (d) False (p. 1151): anorexia nervosa only.
   (e) True (p. 1151): less in intensiveness in hypopituitarism.

160  Neurophysiology of sleep:
(a)  Most adults' sleep–wake cycles are biphasic.
(b)  Orthodox sleep has five stages.
(c)  Slow-wave sleep corresponds with stages 3 and 4 of non-REM sleep.
(d)  The first episode of REM sleep arises approximately 2 hours after a sleep onset.
(e)  As the night progresses the proportion of slow-wave sleep in each cycle increases.

161  The following statements concerning sleep are true:
(a)  Slow-wave sleep is maximal in adolescence.
(b)  Slow-wave sleep is more vulnerable to the effects of age in women.
(c)  High-carbohydrate/low-fat diets have been found to significantly increase REM sleep.
(d)  Heat exposure causes an increase in REM sleep.
(e)  Physical exercise decreases slow-wave sleep.

162  Narcolepsy:
(a)  The cardinal feature is irresistible episodes of sleep at inappropriate times.
(b)  Cataplexy in which there is a complete physical collapse of the patient is rare.
(c)  Sleep paralysis may occur at the point of waking but not at the point of falling asleep.
(d)  Auditory hallucinations are more common than visual hallucinations.
(e)  Narcolepsy is also known as Gelineau's syndrome.

163  The following symptoms are not recognised in narcolepsy:
(a)  Tactile hallucinations.
(b)  Automatic behaviour.
(c)  Disrupted nocturnal sleep.
(d)  Apnoeic episodes in sleep.
(e)  Blurred vision.

164  Epidemiology of narcolepsy:
(a)  Narcolepsy affects 1 in 100,000.
(b)  It is commoner in females.
(c)  Almost 100% of cases are linked with the HLA-DR$_4$ antigen.
(d)  Autosomal recessive inheritance is likely.
(e)  The first symptoms generally occur between the ages of 10 and 20 years.

160 (a) False (p. 1176): monophasic, that is, only one episode of sleep per light–dark cycle.
   (b) False (p. 1177): there are four stages.
   (c) True (p. 1177).
   (d) False (p. 1177): 70 minutes.
   (e) False (p. 1177): diminishes.

161 (a) True (p. 1178): and it declines with advancing years.
   (b) False (p. 1178): in men.
   (c) True (p. 1178): and low-carbohydrate/high-fat diets also.
   (d) False (p. 1180): reduction in REM and slow-wave sleep; exposure to cold decreases REM and stage 2 sleep.
   (e) False (p. 1178): may increase it.

162 (a) True (p. 1195).
   (b) True (p. 1195).
   (c) False (p. 1195): occurs at both.
   (d) False (p. 1195): the reverse is true – visual hallucinations are more common than auditory hypnagogic/hypnopompic hallucinations.
   (e) True (p. 1195).

163 (a) False (p. 1196).
   (b) False (p. 1196).
   (c) False (p. 1196).
   (d) False (p. 1196).
   (e) False (p. 1196).

   Note the negative stem – all the symptoms listed are recognised in narcolepsy.

164 (a) False (p. 1196): 1 in 10 000.
   (b) False (p. 1196): occurs equally in the genders.
   (c) False (p. 1196): almost 100% of cases are linked with the HLA-DR$_2$ antigen.
   (d) False (p. 1196): autosomal dominant with variable penetrance.
   (e) False (p. 1196): between the ages of 15 and 35 years.

165 The features of narcolepsy:

(a) The hallmark is that the individual falls directly into REM latency from wakefulness.
(b) More than 80% of subjects have a mean sleep latency of less than 10 minutes.
(c) Dexamphetamine reduces the risk of cataplexy.
(d) Tricyclic antidepressants can help control sleep paralysis.
(e) Benzodiazepines are contraindicated.

166 Obstructive sleep apnoea:

(a) Frequently presents with excessive daytime sleepiness as the dominant symptom.
(b) Occurs when upper airways patency is lost.
(c) Is rare in adolescence and young adults.
(d) Is commoner in women.
(e) Affects less than 1% of the adult working population.

167 Features of non-organic hypersomnia:

(a) Patients are sometimes difficult to wake and may be abusive on waking.
(b) Symptoms typically start when patients are in their 30s.
(c) Once the condition is established it is incurable and unremitting.
(d) The condition has been associated with viral infections.
(e) A positive family history is rare.

168 Features of the Kleine–Levine syndrome:

(a) Intermittent hypersomnia.
(b) Equal occurrence in the genders.
(c) Hyposexuality.
(d) Polydipsia.
(e) Episodes generally last for hours.

169 Further features of the Kleine–Levine syndrome:

(a) Episodes occur on average twice a year.
(b) It appears to have a familial component.
(c) Initial episode can follow minor infections.
(d) Recurrences dissipate with time and eventually cease.
(e) Stimulants are best avoided.

170 Somnambulism:

(a) Somnambulism occurs in stage 2 slow-wave sleep.
(b) It occurs late in the night.
(c) It affects about 15% of children.
(d) Mental ideation is generally recalled.
(e) It has a higher concordance rate in dizygotic than monozygotic twins.

165 (a) False (p. 1196): REM sleep but not latency.
  (b) False (p. 1197): 5 minutes.
  (c) False (p. 1197): reduces daytime sleepiness – tricyclic antidepressants may help cataplexy.
  (d) True (p. 1197).
  (e) False (p. 1197): may be used if nocturnal sleep disturbance is prominent.

166 (a) True (p. 1197).
  (b) True (p. 1197): in the region of the pharynx.
  (c) True (p. 1198).
  (d) False (p. 1198): men.
  (e) False (p. 1198): 1–5%.

167 (a) False (p. 1200): patients are often difficult to wake and may respond abusively while in a semi-awakened state when aroused, with subsequent amnesia for their behaviour.
  (b) False (p. 1200): late adolescence and young adulthood.
  (c) True (p. 1200).
  (d) True (p. 1200).
  (e) False (p. 1200): there may be a family history.

168 (a) True (p. 1200).
  (b) False (p. 1200): it is more common in young males.
  (c) False (p. 1200): hypersexuality.
  (d) True (p. 1200).
  (e) False (p. 1200): episodes generally last for a few days but may last as long as a month.

169 (a) True (p. 1200).
  (b) False (p. 1202): appears to be non-familial.
  (c) True (p. 1202): can follow minor infections or injury.
  (d) True (p. 1202).
  (e) False (p. 1202): stimulants can be used to combat somnolence.

170 (a) False (p. 1202): stage 4 slow-wave sleep.
  (b) False (p. 1202): usually early in the night.
  (c) True (p. 1202).
  (d) False (p. 1202): not usually recalled.
  (e) False (p. 1203): the reverse is true.

171  Somnambulism may be triggered by:
(a)  Tricyclic antidepressants.
(b)  Beta-blockers.
(c)  Benzodiazepines.
(d)  SSRIs.
(e)  Psychological stress.

172  Night terrors:
(a)  Night terrors affect approximately one-third of children.
(b)  They typically occur in the first one-third of the night.
(c)  Episodes generally last 1–3 minutes.
(d)  There is often limited recall.
(e)  They frequently accompany sleepwalking.

173  Restless leg syndrome:
(a)  The syndrome is primarily a motor disorder.
(b)  It usually occurs unilaterally.
(c)  It rarely occurs in pregnancy.
(d)  Attacks usually occur within 20 minutes of going to bed.
(e)  Symptoms may last from several minutes to several hours.

174  Hypernyctohemeral syndrome:
(a)  The syndrome is also known as the 24-hour sleep–wake syndrome.
(b)  It consists of a steady pattern comprising a 1–2-hour daily delay in sleep onset.
(c)  The sleep–wake cycle is free running.
(d)  It has been well described in congenitally deaf persons.
(e)  It has responded to folate supplements.

175  Shortened REM sleep latency occurs in:
(a)  Depression.
(b)  Schizophrenia.
(c)  Cannabis withdrawal.
(d)  Time zone change syndrome.
(e)  Nocturnal paroxysmal dystonia.

176  Increase in REM sleep occurs:
(a)  In the second half of the night in depression.
(b)  After ECT.
(c)  During carbamazepine therapy.
(d)  After alcohol intoxication.
(e)  After stimulant intoxication.

171 (a) True (p. 1203): certain tricyclic antidepressants.
    (b) True (p. 1203): lipid-soluble beta-blockers.
    (c) True (p. 1203): some benzodiazepines.
    (d) True (p. 1203).
    (e) True (p. 1203).

172 (a) True (p. 1204): at least once.
    (b) True (p. 1204).
    (c) False (p. 1204): 1–10 minutes.
    (d) False (p. 1204): usually complete amnesia for the event.
    (e) False (p. 1204): may occur together.

173 (a) False (p. 1206): primarily a sensory disorder.
    (b) False (p. 1206): usually occurs symmetrically, affecting the lower limbs.
    (c) False (p. 1206).
    (d) True (p. 1206): 5–30 minutes.
    (e) True (p. 1206).

174 (a) False (p. 1211): non-24-hour sleep–wake syndrome.
    (b) True (p. 1211).
    (c) True (p. 1212).
    (d) False (p. 1212): recognised in congenitally blind persons.
    (e) False (p. 1212): has responded well to $B_{12}$ supplements.

175 (a) True (p. 1214).
    (b) True (p. 1216).
    (c) True (p. 1218).
    (d) False (p. 1209): no such description.
    (e) False (p. 1206): no such description.

176 (a) False (p. 1215): in the first half of the night.
    (b) False (p. 1215): ECT suppresses REM sleep.
    (c) False (p. 1215): carbamazepine suppresses REM sleep, as do lithium and other antidepressants.
    (d) False (p. 1217): REM sleep is diminished after alcohol intoxication but increases when alcohol levels fall and is also increased in alcohol withdrawal.
    (e) False (p. 1217): but stimulant intoxication also increases sleep latency and decreases total sleep time and REM and stage 3 and 4 sleep.

177 The effects of alcohol on sleep include:

(a) A decrease in stages 3 and 4 in acute intoxication.
(b) Increased REM in intoxication.
(c) Increased REM in alcohol withdrawal states.
(d) Deficits in the amount of stage 2 sleep following successful alcohol withdrawal in alcohol dependency.
(e) Insomnia.

178 In relation to REM sleep the following are true:

(a) REM rebounds on stimulant withdrawal.
(b) There is increased REM sleep on first exposure to cannabis.
(c) LSD prolongs REM sleep duration.
(d) Benzodiazepines reduce REM.
(e) Tricyclic antidepressants and SSRIs both suppress REM sleep.

179 Monothetic and polythetic diagnosis:

(a) Monothetic diagnoses require all the criteria in the definition to be present.
(b) Monothetic reliability always depends on the reliability of the weakest item.
(c) Polythetic criteria are less robust.
(d) Polythetic diagnoses permit less diagnostic heterogeneity within a class.
(e) Polythetic classification is one in which members of a class share a large proportion of properties but not necessarily the presence of any one property.

180 Determinants of referral to the psychiatrist by a general practitioner include:

(a) Younger age of general practitioner.
(b) Low rate of identification of psychiatric disorder by the general practitioner.
(c) Female patient.
(d) Chronic disorder.
(e) Rural and accessible services.

177 (a)  False (p. 1217): an increase in stages 3 and 4 in acute intoxication.
    (b)  False (p. 1217): a decrease in REM sleep.
    (c)  True (p. 1217).
    (d)  False (p. 1217): stage 4 sleep.
    (e)  True (p. 1217): insomnia is the commonest sleep disorder associated with alcohol.

178 (a)  True (p. 1218).
    (b)  False (p. 1218): on first exposure to cannabis, REM sleep duration is reduced, but it returns to normal with regular use.
    (c)  True (p. 1218).
    (d)  True (p. 1219).
    (e)  True (p. 1220): also true for MAOIs, lithium and carbamazepine.

179 (a)  True (p. 1241).
    (b)  True (p. 1241).
    (c)  False (p. 1241): polythetic criteria are more robust.
    (d)  False (p. 1241): polythetic diagnoses permit more diagnostic heterogeneity within a class.
    (e)  True (p. 1241).

180 (a)  False (p. 1349): older age of general practitioner.
    (b)  False (p. 1349): high rate of identification of psychiatric disorder by the general practitioner.
    (c)  False (p. 1349): male patient.
    (d)  True (p. 1349): duration over 1 year.
    (e)  False (p. 1349): urban and accessible.

# The Psychiatry of Learning Disabilities

1    The following statements are true with respect to learning disabilities:
(a)    Mild intellectual impairment corresponds to an IQ of 55–69.
(b)    There is geographical variation in the prevalence of severe intellectual impairment among similar birth cohorts.
(c)    Temporal variation in the prevalence of severe intellectual impairment does not exist in successive birth cohorts in the same community.
(d)    There is increased survival at all ages among those with severe learning impairment.
(e)    There are no consistent patterns in the gender ratio.

2    Features of Down's syndrome include:
(a)    Approximately 95% are due to disjunction of chromosome 21.
(b)    5% show mosaicism.
(c)    Up to 20% of non-disjunctions are of paternal origin.
(d)    IQ generally is less than 35.
(e)    Foetuses with Down's syndrome have a very high mortality late in gestation.

3    Features of the fragile X syndrome:
(a)    Fragile X is usually associated with a reduction in size of a repeat sequence near the promoter of a gene called FMR1.
(b)    The responsible gene is on the short arm of the X chromosome at Xp27.
(c)    Multiple repeats of a CGG trinucleotide triplet lead to methylation and silencing of the gene.
(d)    Approximately 80% of affected boys have an IQ of less than 50.
(e)    One-third of males with fragile X have epileptic seizures.

4    Diagnostic rating scales used in learning disability:
(a)    The Aberrant Behaviour Checklist has seven sub-scales.
(b)    The Diagnostic Assessment Scale for the Severely Handicapped is a multidimensional instrument used to assess severity of symptoms.
(c)    The Reiss Screen for maladaptive behaviour is usually completed by a clinician.
(d)    The Psychopathology Inventory for Mentally Retarded Adults can be self-reported or reported by a third party.
(e)    The Psychiatric Assessment Scale for Adults with Developmental Disability is derived from the Present State Examination.

1   (a)  False (p. 17): IQ of 50–69.
    (b)  True (p. 23).
    (c)  False (p. 23): temporal variation exists.
    (d)  True (p. 23).
    (e)  True (p. 23).

2   (a)  False (pp. 32–33): non-disjunction.
    (b)  False (p. 33): now suggested to be 2–4% who show mosaicism; 3–5% are familial due to translocation.
    (c)  False (p. 33): should read only 5% maximum. (The figures originally published are now out of date.)
    (d)  False (p. 33): 20–55.
    (e)  False (p. 33): early in gestation.

3   (a)  False (p. 33): expansion in the gene called FMRI.
    (b)  False (p. 33): Xq27.
    (c)  True (p. 33).
    (d)  False (p. 33): 80% have an IQ of less than 70.
    (e)  False (p. 36): 20%.

4   (a)  False (p. 58): it has five sub-scales – irritability, agitation and crying; lethargy and social withdrawal; stereotypical behaviour; hyperactivity and non-compliance; and inappropriate speech.
    (b)  True (p. 58).
    (c)  False (p. 38): it is usually completed by the carer, teacher or other person who knows the subject well.
    (d)  True (p. 58).
    (e)  True (p. 59).

5   The following conditions are generally associated with at least severe learning disability:
(a)   Cornelia de Lange syndrome.
(b)   Lesch–Nyhan syndrome.
(c)   Prader–Willi syndrome.
(d)   Rett's syndrome.
(e)   Neurofibromatosis.

6   The following are true with regard to mode of inheritance:
(a)   Duchenne's muscular dystrophy is X-linked recessive at Xp21.
(b)   Female carriers of Lesch–Nyhan are mosaic for the condition due to random inactivation of the X chromosome.
(c)   Phenylketonuria (PKU) incidence shows variation across ethnic groups.
(d)   Prader–Willi syndrome derives from a lack of maternal 15q.
(e)   Neurofibromatosis is autosomal dominant.

7   Features of the fragile X syndrome include:
(a)   Cluttered speech.
(b)   High arched feet.
(c)   Short-term memory deficits.
(d)   Multiple copies of a CGG trinucleotide repeat expand down generations particularly when passed through a male meiosis.
(e)   Testicular enlargement which occurs only post-pubertally.

8   The somatic phenotype of Prader–Willi syndrome includes:
(a)   Mild learning disability.
(b)   Frequent spinal deformities.
(c)   Hypogonadism.
(d)   Small extremities.
(e)   Non-food-related belligerence.

9   Features of Angelman's syndrome include:
(a)   A small deletion of a differentially imprinted region on the short arm of the paternal chromosome 15.
(b)   Mild to moderate learning disability.
(c)   Pica.
(d)   Sleep disturbance.
(e)   Attention deficit syndrome.

5  (a) True (p. 64): throughout the ability range but majority severe to profound.
   (b) False (p. 64): mild to moderate learning disability.
   (c) False (p. 64): borderline to moderate learning disability.
   (d) True (p. 64): severe to profound.
   (e) False (p. 64): low average ability and only 10% have significant learning disability.

6  (a) True (p. 64).
   (b) True (p. 64): also Lesch–Nyhan is nearly always due to a sporadic mutation in the HPRT gene at Xq26–27.
   (c) True (p. 64): PKU is autosomal recessive with mutations in the PAH gene at 12q22–24.
   (d) False (p. 64): paternal 15q.
   (e) True (p. 64): but now known to be several conditions.

7  (a) True (p. 69): fast and garbled with repetitive quality and articulation problems.
   (b) False (p. 69): they have flat feet and a high arched palate.
   (c) True (p. 69).
   (d) False (p. 68): this would be true if transmitted through females.
   (e) False (p. 69): also known to occur prepubertally.

8  (a) True (p. 70).
   (b) True (p. 70).
   (c) True (p. 70).
   (d) True (p. 70).
   (e) False (p. 71): this is a behavioural phenotype.

   Note. The somatic phenotype also includes obesity, short stature and poor muscle tone; pervasive and puzzling dystrophy, connective tissue defects, increased bleeding problems and friable bones; sleep apnoea with daytime drowsiness, expressive language disorder compounded by poor articulation. Visual perception skills may be a particular strength and extend to hyperlexia. Genetically, there is a lack of paternal 15 (q11–13 ). Initially the hypotonia leads to feeding difficulties and poor weight gain, but an insatiable hunger drive develops from about 3 years of age. This, coupled with a defective sense of satiety, soon leads to obesity. There is also a lower metabolic rate. Outbursts of violent temper occur. There is a higher incidence of psychiatric disturbance, with incessant skin picking, and compulsive or anxiety neurosis.

9  (a) False (p. 71): the child lacks a maternal contribution to chromosome 15.
   (b) False (p. 71): severe learning disability.
   (c) True (p. 71).
   (d) True (p. 71).
   (e) True (p. 71): also has a characteristic facies, ataxic and jerky movements and an affectionate and cheerful disposition ('happy puppet').

10   Features of Lesch–Nyhan syndrome include:
(a)   Non-compulsive self-mutilation.
(b)   Exclusivity to females.
(c)   Failure of secondary sexual development.
(d)   Death in early adulthood from liver failure.
(e)   Hypertonia.

11   Features of Williams syndrome include:
(a)   Mitral valve prolapse.
(b)   Severe learning disability.
(c)   Joint laxity.
(d)   Good verbal ability in contrast to learning disability.
(e)   Hypersensitivity to sound.

12   Rett's syndrome:
(a)   The syndrome occurs only in females.
(b)   It is probably X-linked recessive.
(c)   Typically there is autistic withdrawal.
(d)   The first 6–18 months are normal developmentally.
(e)   Hypotonicity.

13   The following psychiatric symptoms are more prevalent in children
     with an IQ of less than 70 than among those with an IQ of over 70:
(a)   Anxiety and phobic states.
(b)   Depressive syndromes.
(c)   Asperger's syndrome.
(d)   Anorexia nervosa.
(e)   Pica.

10  (a)  False (p. 73): compulsive self-mutilation, which is distressing to these children, who prefer imposed restraint.
   (b)  False (p. 73): almost exclusive to males – it is an X-linked condition.
   (c)  True (p. 73).
   (d)  False (p. 73): respiratory or renal failure is generally the cause of death.
   (e)  True (p. 73): hypotonic initially followed by hypertonia.

   Note. Additional features include: normal development in early infancy except for orange uricosuric sand in the nappy; hypotonia followed by spastic choreo-athetosis, dysphagia and dysarthria, with seizures in about 50%; specific or moderate learning difficulties. There is a deficiency of hypoxanthine-guanine phosphoribosyl transferase (HPRT), an enzyme involved in purine metabolism. Uric acid is released in excess but allopurinol yields no psychological benefit, even though it reduces uric acid levels.

11  (a)  True (pp. 72–73): also aortic stenosis.
   (b)  False (p. 73): mild to moderate learning disability.
   (c)  False (p. 74): joint contractures with progressive joint limitation, kyphosis and scoliosis.
   (d)  True (p. 73).
   (e)  True (p. 73).

   Note. Other features include: 'elfin' facies, cardiovascular complications including hypertension, valvular lesions, and a variety of urinary and gastrointestinal problems. Calcium levels may be raised, particularly in infancy.

12  (a)  False (p. 74): it may be a lethal disorder in boys.
   (b)  False (p. 75): X-linked dominant.
   (c)  True (p. 74).
   (d)  True (p. 74): near normal or normal.
   (e)  False (p. 74): spasticity.

   Note. After 6–18 months of nearly normal development, the child starts to dement and head growth slows. Typically there is an autistic withdrawal accompanied by seizures, stereotypical movements (notably hand-wringing), agitation, hyperventilation and breath-holding. Truncal ataxia, spasticity and dystonia follow. Depression and anxiety are frequent, with self-injury and panic when threatened.

13  (a)  False (p. 83).
   (b)  False (p. 83).
   (c)  False (p. 83).
   (d)  False (p. 83): likewise school refusal, socialised conduct disorder, schizophrenia and bulimia are more prevalent among those with an IQ of over 70.
   (e)  True (p. 83): likewise autistic traits, hyperkinesis, uncontrolled rage, self-injury, sleep disturbances and unsocialised conduct disorder are more prevalent among those with an IQ of under 70.

14 The Checklist for Autism in Toddlers (CHAT) includes:

(a) Predictors of autism at 36 months.
(b) An item relating to lack of pretend play.
(c) An item relating to lack of proto-declarative pointing.
(d) An item relating to resistance to change.
(e) An item relating to lack of joint attention.

15 In relation to autism:

(a) Gross pathology in the cerebellar vermis has been described.
(b) Enlargement of lateral and third ventricle has been described.
(c) Platelet serotonin has been shown to be consistently elevated in 30% of sufferers.
(d) Low levels of dopa hydroxylase have been found in probands.
(e) Increased Purkinje cell counts have been described.

16 Alzheimer's disease and Down's syndrome:

(a) The pathological brain changes seen in the general population differ from those seen in Down's syndrome.
(b) Reduced levels of cytoplasmic superoxide dismutase (SOD) in Down's syndrome may contribute to accelerated ageing.
(c) Personality change is an infrequent presenting symptom.
(d) Epilepsy developing for the first time in those with Down's syndrome aged over 35 years is usually associated with Alzheimer's disease.
(e) Macrocytosis due to abnormal erythrocyte membrane components is frequently seen in people with Down's syndrome and dementia.

17 Behavioural interventions:

(a) Procedures for differentially reinforcing alternative behaviours arrange for the individual to receive additional programmed reinforcers while engaged in target behaviour.
(b) Aversive therapy pairs the inappropriate discrimination with overt aversive stimuli.
(c) Orgasmic reconditioning involves the use of the inappropriate discrimination stimuli to initiate sexual activity but involves a switch to appropriate discrimination stimuli before orgasm.
(d) Escape extinction is the extinction of behaviours maintained by negative reinforcement.
(e) Response cost is the removal of specific positive reinforcers following an episode of challenging behaviour.

18 The following are average normal ages of milestones of speech and language acquisition:

(a) Two-word utterances at 1 year.
(b) Fifty-word lexicon at 2.5 years.
(c) Plurals established at 2 years.
(d) Telegrammatic speech at 3 years.
(e) 'How' and 'why' questions emerge at 4.5 years.

14  (a) False (p. 106): 30 months.
    (b) True (p. 107).
    (c) True (p. 107).
    (d) False (p. 106): this is not a CHAT item but it is a feature of autism.
    (e) True (p. 106).

15  (a) False (p. 116): little evidence of gross pathology.
    (b) True (p. 116).
    (c) True (p. 117).
    (d) True (p. 117): also true for first-degree relatives.
    (e) False (p. 116): decreased Purkinje cell counts in cerebellar vermis.

16  (a) False (p. 140): the pathological changes are the same.
    (b) False (p. 141): elevated levels of SOD.
    (c) False (p. 141): it is a frequent presenting symptom.
    (d) True (p. 142).
    (e) True (p. 142): in the presence of normal vitamin $B_{12}$ and folic acid levels.

17  (a) True (p. 171).
    (b) True (p. 173): for example noxious smells and electric shocks.
    (c) True (p. 173).
    (d) True (p. 174): by prevention of escape from the aversive stimuli.
    (e) True (p. 174): for example fines.

18  (a) False (p. 180): 18 months.
    (b) True (p. 180).
    (c) False (p. 180): 3 years.
    (d) False (p. 180): 20 months.
    (e) False (p. 180): 3.5 years.

19  Epilepsy and learning disability:
(a)  In those with an IQ of 50–75 the rate of epilepsy is 20%.
(b)  Treatment of epilepsy may lower IQ.
(c)  Sturge–Weber syndrome results in reduced IQ and epilepsy.
(d)  The commonest cause of most epilepsy in people with learning disability is developmental.
(e)  Seizures rarely reduce IQ.

20  The following are classified as generalised seizures:
(a)  Absence seizures.
(b)  Myoclonic seizures.
(c)  Atonic seizures.
(d)  'Jacksonian' seizures.
(e)  'Psychomotor' attacks.

21  Features of West syndrome:
(a)  Flexor and extensor myoclonic spasms.
(b)  Moderate learning disability.
(c)  Onset between 1 and 2 years.
(d)  Burst suppression on electroencephalography (EEG).
(e)  Tuberose sclerosis as a common cause.

22  Causes of West syndrome include:
(a)  Leucodystrophy.
(b)  Perinatal hypoxia.
(c)  Down's syndrome.
(d)  Inborn errors of metabolism.
(e)  Prenatal infections.

23  The following types of seizures occur in Lennox–Gastaut syndrome:
(a)  Atypical absences.
(b)  Tonic seizures.
(c)  Atonic seizures.
(d)  Myoclonic seizures.
(e)  Status epilepticus.

24  Features of Lennox–Gastaut syndrome:
(a)  EEG shows ictal diffuse slow spike and wave changes.
(b)  Age of onset is over 1 year.
(c)  Males and females are equally affected.
(d)  It may be preceded by West's syndrome.
(e)  Seizures are usually clonic initially.

19  (a)  False (p. 223): the rate is 5%. Among those with an IQ of less than
         50 it is 30% and among those with an IQ of less than 20 it is 50%.
    (b)  True (p. 224): for example surgery and sedating drugs.
    (c)  True (p. 224): also lipidosis and tuberose sclerosis, disintegrative
         psychosis.
    (d)  True (p. 224).
    (e)  True (p. 224).

20  (a)  True (p. 227).
    (b)  True (p. 227).
    (c)  True (p. 227): 'drop attacks'.
    (d)  False (p. 227): simple partial seizures.
    (e)  False (p. 227): complex partial seizures with impaired consciousness
         at onset either alone or with automatisms.

21  (a)  True (p. 233): flexor (salaam) and extensor myoclonic spasms of
         the neck, trunk and limbs.
    (b)  False (p. 233): severe learning disability.
    (c)  False (p. 233): less than 1 year – usually 3–7 months.
    (d)  False (p. 233): hypsarrhythmia – an EEG pattern of a chaotic mixture
         of high-amplitude slow waves with variable spikes and sharp waves.
    (e)  True (p. 233).

22  (a)  True (p. 233).
    (b)  True (p. 233).
    (c)  True (p. 233).
    (d)  True (p. 233).
    (e)  True (p. 233).

         Note. Prognosis is poor and depends on the underlying condition. Only 20%
         will make a complete recovery.

23  (a)  True (p. 234).
    (b)  True (p. 234): usually tonic initially; they may be focal or axial.
    (c)  True (p. 234).
    (d)  True (p. 234).
    (e)  True (p. 234).

24  (a)  False (p. 234): EEG shows inter-ictal diffuse slow spike and wave
         changes. Ictal EEG depends on the form of seizure.
    (b)  True (p. 234): usually between 3 and 5 years of age.
    (c)  False (p. 234): male predominance.
    (d)  True (p. 234).
    (e)  False (p. 234): seizures are usually tonic initially.

# Basic Neurosciences

1   Brain structure:
(a)   The brain-stem links the forebrain and hindbrain.
(b)   The tectum forms the roof of the forebrain.
(c)   The superior cerebellar peduncle attaches the cerebellum to the pons.
(d)   The tegmentum lies between the tectum and the cerebral peduncles.
(e)   The Rolandic fissure delineates temporal and parietal regions.

2   The blood supply to the brain:
(a)   The basilar artery runs along the midline of the pons.
(b)   The medulla is supplied by branches of the posterior inferior cerebellar arteries.
(c)   The external carotid artery divides to form the middle cerebral and anterior cerebral arteries.
(d)   The internal capsule is supplied by the circle of Willis.
(e)   The middle cerebral artery supplies Broca's and Wernicke's areas.

3   Ventricles:
(a)   The body of the lateral ventricle is situated immediately above the corpus callosum.
(b)   The septum pallidum separates the two lateral ventricles.
(c)   The third ventricle lies between the thalamus and the hypothalamus.
(d)   The fourth ventricle lies above the pons.
(e)   The aqueduct of Sylvius links the third and lateral ventricles.

4   Cerbrospinal fluid (CSF):
(a)   CSF is secreted by choroid plexus.
(b)   It is produced at a rate of 300 ml a day.
(c)   It is almost protein free.
(d)   It passes into the subarachnoid space via recesses in the third ventricle.
(e)   Obstruction to its circulation commonly occurs within lateral ventricles.

5   The following cranial nerves have only a sensory component:
(a)   Vestibulocochlear.
(b)   Glossopharyngeal.
(c)   Optic.
(d)   Vagus.
(e)   Olfactory.

1   (a)  False (p. 2): the brain-stem links the forebrain and spinal cord. The
         hindbrain comprises the brain-stem and cerebellum.
    (b)  False (p. 2): the tectum forms the roof of the midbrain.
    (c)  False (p. 2): the middle cerebellar peduncle attaches the cerebellum
         to the pons.
    (d)  True (p. 2).
    (e)  False (p. 2): the Rolandic fissure delineates the frontal and parietal
         regions; it is also known as the central sulcus.

2   (a)  True (p. 4): formed by vertebral arteries.
    (b)  True (p. 4): and the anterior spinal arteries.
    (c)  False (p. 5): the internal carotid divides to form the middle cerebral
         and anterior cerebral arteries.
    (d)  True (p. 5).
    (e)  True (p. 5).

3   (a)  False (p. 7): immediately below the corpus callosum.
    (b)  False (p. 7): the septum pellucidum separates the two lateral ventricles.
    (c)  True (p. 7).
    (d)  True (p. 7): and also below the cerebellum.
    (e)  True (p. 7): the aqueduct of Sylvius links the third and fourth
         ventricles.

4   (a)  True (p. 7).
    (b)  True (p. 7).
    (c)  True (p. 7).
    (d)  False (p. 7): CSF passes into the subarachnoid space via recesses in
         the fourth ventricle – the foramena of Luschka and Magendie.
    (e)  False (p. 8): obstruction to its circulation commonly occurs within
         the third or fourth ventricle.

5   (a)  True (p. 9).
    (b)  False (p. 9): the glossopharyngeal nerve has motor and autonomic
         components in addition to sensory components (taste and general
         sensation from posterior tongue and upper larynx). The motor
         component regulates swallowing, and raises the larynx and pharynx.
         Autonomic function is in the form of salivation from the parotid gland.
    (c)  True (p. 9).
    (d)  False (p. 9): the vagus nerve has a motor component (swallowing
         and phonation). It also has an autonomic component which controls
         the heart, stomach and other thoracic and abdominal viscera.
    (e)  True (p. 9).

6    The following cranial nerves have only a motor component:
(a)  Occulomotor.
(b)  Abducent.
(c)  Accessory.
(d)  Glossopharyngeal.
(e)  Vagus.

7    The following cranial nerves have motor, sensory and autonomic components:
(a)  Occulomotor.
(b)  Facial.
(c)  Glossopharyngeal.
(d)  Vagus.
(e)  Trigeminal.

8    Features of the facial nerve include:
(a)  Supplies taste to the anterior third of the tongue.
(b)  Carries sensation from the back of the internal ear.
(c)  Elevates the hyoid bone.
(d)  Tenses the stapes.
(e)  Innervation of the parotid and submandibular glands.

9    Salivation is dependent on the following cranial nerves:
(a)  Facial.
(b)  Trigeminal.
(c)  Vagus.
(d)  Glossopharyngeal.
(e)  Hypoglossal.

10   Somaesthesia:
(a)  Dermatones do not correspond with the distribution of peripheral nerves.
(b)  The dorsal columns and medial lemniscus include pathways for limb position.
(c)  The gracile and cuneate columns form the dorsal columns.
(d)  Information from receptors serving pain and temperature reach the spinal cord via fast myelinated fibres.
(e)  Pain and pressure travel in anterior spinothalamic tracts.

6   (a)  False (p. 9): also autonomic (focusing and pupillary constriction).
    (b)  True (p. 9).
    (c)  True (p. 9).
    (d)  False (p. 9): sensory, motor and autonomic.
    (e)  False (p. 9): sensory, motor and autonomic.

    Note. Cranial nerves with solely a motor component are trochlear, abducent, accessory and hypoglossal.

7   (a)  False (p. 9): it has motor and autonomic components.
    (b)  True (p. 9).
    (c)  True (p. 9).
    (d)  True (p. 9).
    (e)  False (p. 9): sensory and motor only.

8   (a)  False (p. 9): anterior two-thirds.
    (b)  False (p. 9): sensation from back of the external ear.
    (c)  True (p. 9).
    (d)  True (p. 9).
    (e)  False (p. 9): it is an autonomic component that controls lacrimation and salivation to the sublingual and submandibular glands.

9   (a)  True (p. 9): sublingual and submandibular.
    (b)  False (p. 9).
    (c)  False (p. 9).
    (d)  True (p. 9): parotid.
    (e)  False (p. 9).

10  (a)  True (p. 11): cutaneous distribution of a spinal nerve is known as its dermatone.
    (b)  True (p. 11)): the dorsal columns and medial lemniscus are pathways for two-point discrimination, limb position and vibration sense.
    (c)  True (p. 11).
    (d)  False (p. 13): information from receptors serving diffuse touch, pressure, pain and temperature reaches the spinal cord via slow-conducting C and A delta fibres in the spinothalamic tracts, whose cell bodies lie in the dorsal root ganglia.
    (e)  False (p. 14): touch and pressure travel in the anterior spinothalamic tract; pain and temperature travel in the lateral spinothalamic tract.

11   The following are true with reference to dissociation of sensation:
(a)   The spinothalamic and dorsal column systems diverge at the dorsal horn.
(b)   The spinothalamic tracts decussate a little below their segment of origin in the spinal cord.
(c)   The dorsal column pathway does not cross until the medulla.
(d)   Brown–Séquard syndrome involves contralateral loss of pain and temperature and ipsilateral two-point discrimination loss.
(e)   If sensory loss affects spinothalamic and dorsal column sensation equally, the lesion is likely to be outside the central nervous system (CNS).

12   The visual pathways:
(a)   Axons serving the temporal visual fields cross the midline in the optic chiasm.
(b)   The optic tracts terminate in the lateral geniculate body.
(c)   Damage to an optic nerve causes partial or total blindness in the contralateral eye.
(d)   Lesions affecting the midline of the optic chiasm are associated with hemianopia affecting nasal fields.
(e)   Lesions behind the chiasm result in homonymous defects.

13   The following statements are true with reference to visual pathways:
(a)   The input to the inferior colliculus serves as the afferent limb for the visual avoidance reflexes.
(b)   Fibres which relay in the pretectal area mediate the pupillary light reflex.
(c)   Sympathetic fibres of the oculomotor nerve innervate the constrictor pupillae within the eye.
(d)   'Consensual response' relies on the projection of the pretectal area to the contralateral Edinger–Westphal nucleus.
(e)   Horner's syndrome results from parasympathetic damage.

14   The auditory pathway is dependent on the following structures:
(a)   Trapezoid body.
(b)   Superior olivary nucleus.
(c)   Medial lemniscus.
(d)   Lateral geniculate body.
(e)   Heschl's gyrus.

11  (a)  True  (p. 14): and reconverge at the thalamus.
    (b)  False (p. 14): the spinothalamic and dorsal column systems diverge at the dorsal horn and reconverge at the thalamus.
    (c)  True  (p. 14).
    (d)  True  (p. 14): extensive damage in one-half of the spinal cord can give rise to loss of pain and temperature in dermatomes below and contralateral to the lesion, but to loss of two-point discrimination ipsilaterally.
    (e)  True  (p. 14): or above the thalamus.

12  (a)  True  (p. 16): axons which originate in the nasal half of each retina and which therefore serve the temporal visual fields cross the midline in the optic chiasm; those which originate in the temporal half of each retina serving the nasal visual fields remain in the lateral position in the chiasm and do not cross.
    (b)  True  (p. 16).
    (c)  False (p. 16): causes partial or total blindness in the ipsilateral eye.
    (d)  False (pp. 16–17): are associated with scotomata or even hemianopia affecting temporal fields. Some pituitary tumours and hypothalamic tumours can do this.
    (e)  True  (p. 17): that is, they affect equivalent parts of the field of both eyes. When the lesion involves Meyer's loop, only the upper part of the contralateral field is affected. Thus homonymous field defects in an upper quadrant of the field of the visual field may provide an early indication of disorder in the contralateral temporal lobe.

13  (a)  False (p. 18): it is the input to the superior colliculus which serves as the afferent limb for the visual avoidance reflexes, which are the blinks and postural movements evoked by sudden changes in brightness or by approaching visual stimuli.
    (b)  True  (p. 18): axons pass from the pretectal area to the para-sympathetic Edinger–Westphal nucleus of each oculomotor nerve; parasympathetic fibres of the oculomotor nerve innervate the constrictor pupillae within the eye.
    (c)  False (p. 18): parasympathetic.
    (d)  True  (p. 18): constriction of the contralateral pupil is known as the 'consensual response'.
    (e)  False (p. 19): damage to sympathetic fibres, which results in a fixed constricted pupil, due to the unopposed action of the oculomotor nerve.

14  (a)  True  (p. 20).
    (b)  True  (p. 20).
    (c)  False (p. 20): lateral lemniscus.
    (d)  False (p. 20): medial geniculate body.
    (e)  True  (p. 20): Heschl's gyrus is the auditory cortex.

15 The following are involved in the visual pathway:
(a) Myer's loop.
(b) Medial geniculate body.
(c) Tegmentum.
(d) Inferior colliculus.
(e) Corona radiata.

16 The following are true statements:
(a) Unilateral lesions of Heschl's gyrus result in unilateral deafness.
(b) The predominance of the crossed pathway can be demonstrated by the 'dichotic listening' test.
(c) Words presented to the right ear are more accurately reported than those presented simultaneously to the left ear.
(d) Focal lesions in the cortex seldom give rise to auditory signs to aid localisation.
(e) The inferior colliculus is the origin of pathways involved in postural reflexes in response to sudden loud noises.

17 Lesions in the corpus striatum are associated with:
(a) Athetosis.
(b) Huntington's chorea.
(c) Dystonia.
(d) Hemiballismus.
(e) Parkinson's disease.

18 The following effects are associated with lesions to the right hemisphere:
(a) Receptive amusia.
(b) Contralateral neglect.
(c) Gerstmann's syndrome.
(d) Achromatopsia.
(e) Broca's aphasia.

19 The following effects are associated with lesions to the left hemisphere:
(a) Alexia without agraphia.
(b) Alexia with agraphia.
(c) Agraphia without alexia.
(d) Prosopagnosia.
(e) Constructional apraxia.

15  (a)  True (p. 17): Myer's loop is part of the optic radiation.
    (b)  False (p. 17): lateral geniculate body.
    (c)  False (p. 17).
    (d)  False (p. 20): the inferior colliculus is involved in the auditory pathway.
    (e)  True (p. 16).

16  (a)  False (p. 20): each auditory cortex (Heschl's gyrus) receives information from both ears.
    (b)  True (p. 21): in competitive stimulation of the ears ('dichotic listening'), words presented to the right ear are more accurately reported than those presented simultaneously to the left ear, since the speech areas are normally situated in the left hemisphere.
    (c)  True (p. 21).
    (d)  True (p. 21): as a result of the bilateral projection to the cortex.
    (e)  True (p. 21): sudden loud sounds evoke postural reflexes which may involve avoidance or orientation towards the source; the inferior colliculus is the origin of the tectospinal and tectobulbar pathways which elicit the necessary responses in motor neurons.

17  (a)  True (p. 26).
    (b)  True (p. 26).
    (c)  True (p. 26).
    (d)  False (p. 26): subthalamic lesion.
    (e)  False (p. 26): lesions in the substantia nigra.

18  (a)  True (p. 30): this is the inability to appreciate music.
    (b)  True (p. 30).
    (c)  False (p. 30): left hemisphere.
    (d)  True (p. 30): right or bilateral.
    (e)  False (p. 30): left hemisphere.

    Note. Right hemisphere lesions may also produce: constructional apraxia, colour agnosia, prosopagnosia (right or bilateral), anosognosia, autotopagnosia, visual spatial agnosia.

19  (a)  True (p. 30).
    (b)  True (p. 30).
    (c)  True (p. 30).
    (d)  False (p. 30): right or bilateral.
    (e)  False (p. 30): right hemisphere.

    Note. Left hemisphere lesions may also produce: colour anomia without aphasia, Gerstmann's syndrome, Broca's aphasia, Wernicke's aphasia, acalculia.

20  Damage to the right parietal lobe produces disorders of:
(a)  Body image.
(b)  Anosognosia.
(c)  Autopagnosia.
(d)  Ability to read Braille.
(e)  Dressing apraxia.

21  Right temporal area damage may result in:
(a)  A reduction of score on the Seashore Musical Aptitude test.
(b)  Receptive amusia.
(c)  Difficulty distinguishing complex abstract shapes.
(d)  Difficulty solving visual problems in three-dimensional space.
(e)  Failure to attend to appearance.

22  Components of the limbic system include:
(a)  Cingulate gyrus.
(b)  Posterior nucleus of the thalamus.
(c)  Amygdala.
(d)  Septal nuclei.
(e)  Dorsal longitudinal fasciculus.

23  The major neurotransmitters in the basal ganglia and their interconnections are:
(a)  Dopamine.
(b)  Gamma-aminobutyric acid (GABA).
(c)  Acetylcholine.
(d)  Serotonin (5-hydroxytryptamine; 5-HT).
(e)  Glutamate.

24  The startle response:
(a)  Is dependent on an intact reticular formation.
(b)  Is absent in decerebrate animals.
(c)  Is extensor in all four limbs.
(d)  Is usually followed by a motionless state.
(e)  Is a primitive response.

20  (a)  True (p. 32).
    (b)  True (p. 32): this is failure to acknowledge illness.
    (c)  True (p. 32): this is failure to recognise parts of the body as self.
    (d)  True (p. 32).
    (e)  True (p. 32).

    Note. In addition, neglect (failure to attend to hygiene and appearance) and spatial disorientation.

21  (a)  True (p. 32).
    (b)  True (p. 32).
    (c)  False (p. 32): a feature of damage to the right occipital lobe.
    (d)  False (p. 32): a feature of damage to the right occipital lobe.
    (e)  False (p. 32): a feature of damage to the right parietal lobe.

22  (a)  True (p. 33): connected to the hippocampus by the cingulum; it also has connections to the anterior nucleus of the thalamus and the motor systems via basal ganglia and frontal cortex.
    (b)  False (p. 33): anterior nucleus of the thalamus.
    (c)  True (p. 33): linked to the hypothalamus by the stria terminalis.
    (d)  True (p. 33).
    (e)  False (p. 33): links the hypothalamus with the autonomic nervous system.

    Note. In addition, the hippocampus and the mammillary bodies are parts of the limbic system.

23  (a)  True (p. 62): nigrostriatal pathway, which produces inhibitory postsynaptic potentials in neostriatal interneurons; this pathway becomes progressively impaired in Parkinson's disease.
    (b)  True (p. 62): found in many interneurons within the neostriatum and within neurons projecting from the caudate and putamen to globus pallidus and to substantia nigra; often GABA may be co-localised with neuropeptides such as enkephalin or substance P.
    (c)  True (p. 62): in giant aspiny interneurons within the neostriatum, and which exert a very powerful influence on the GABA-containing interneurons, so disinhibiting the circuit.
    (d)  True (p. 62): Raphe neurons.
    (e)  True (p. 62): input pathway from cortex to neostriatum. Similarly true for aspartate.

24  (a)  True (p. 69).
    (b)  False (p. 69): occurs in decerebrate animals.
    (c)  False (p. 69): the immediate response is flexor in all four limbs.
    (d)  False (p. 69): the response is usually followed by other movements.
    (e)  True (p. 69).

25 The following are excitatory amino acids:
(a) Glycine.
(b) GABA.
(c) Glutamic acid.
(d) Acetylcholine.
(e) N-methyl-D-aspartate (NMDA).

26 With regard to excitatory amino acids the following are true:
(a) GABA is the predominant excitatory amino acid.
(b) NMDA is an excitatory amino acid receptor.
(c) Glutamate is the predominant sensory transmitter in the CNS.
(d) Dizocilpine injected into the hippocampus enhances maze learning in rats.
(e) Excitatory amino acid agonists are potent anticonvulsants in animal models.

27 GABA:
(a) An estimated 40% of all brain synapses use it.
(b) GABA is derived from an excitatory amino acid.
(c) Inhibitors of glutamic acid decarboxylase cause seizures.
(d) GABA is tonically active.
(e) Benzodiazepines and barbiturates modulate GABA indirectly.

28 Acetylcholine:
(a) Is the primary excitatory transmitter at the neuromuscular junction.
(b) Neuronal stores of acetylcholine are depleted by hemicholinium.
(c) In Alzheimer's disease there is marked loss of choline acetyltransferase.
(d) REM sleep can be induced by giving cholinergic agonists.
(e) Anticholinergic agents are profoundly amnestic.

29 With reference to dopamine the following statements are true:
(a) Dopamine-beta-hydroxylase is the rate-limiting step in the synthesis of the catecholamines.
(b) Brain dopamine derives from cell bodies in the midbrain.
(c) Extrapyramidal side-effects emerge with greater than 60% receptor blockade.
(d) Clozapine has a higher ratio of $5\text{-HT}_2:D_2$ receptor blocking ability than conventional neuroleptics.
(e) Bromocryptine is a selective dopamine receptor antagonist.

25   (a)  False (p. 84): it is an inhibitory amino acid.
     (b)  False (p. 84): it is an inhibitory amino acid.
     (c)  True (p. 81).
     (d)  False (p. 90): it is an excitatory transmitter.
     (e)  False (p. 81): it is an excitatory amino acid receptor.

> Note. The important inhibitory amino acids are GABA and glycine. Excitatory amino acids are glutamic acid, aspartate and homocysteine.

26   (a)  False (p. 81): glutamate; GABA is a major inhibitory amino acid.
     (b)  True (p. 81): also AMPA, kainate.
     (c)  True (p. 82).
     (d)  False (p. 83): long-term potentiation is blocked by both competitive and non-competitive antagonists, and these classes of drugs have profound amnestic properties, so that focal injections of dizocilpine into the hippocampus can prevent spatial (maze) learning in rats.
     (e)  False (p. 83): excitatory amino acid antagonists are potent anti-convulsants, as overactivity of excitatory amino acid input is a possible cause of epilepsy. Unfortunately their ability to block memory and produce dissociative states prevents their clinical use.

27   (a)  True (p. 84).
     (b)  True (p. 84): glutamate.
     (c)  True (p. 84).
     (d)  True (p. 84).
     (e)  True (p. 87): benzodiazepine agonists act indirectly to augment GABA; in the absence of GABA they have no action on chloride flux, whereas if GABA is present they make it more efficacious. The barbiturates also modulate GABA indirectly, but at higher concentrations they have direct channel-opening properties, which probably explains their dangerousness in overdose.

28   (a)  True (p. 90): also in preganglionic autonomic nerves.
     (b)  True (p. 90): hemicholinium blocks choline uptake.
     (c)  True (p. 90).
     (d)  True (p. 93): and delayed by muscarinic receptor antagonists.
     (e)  True (p. 92): for example scopolamine.

29   (a)  False (p. 94): tyrosine hydroxylase is the rate-limiting step in the synthesis of the catecholamines.
     (b)  True (p. 95): the largest nucleus being the substantia nigra. Other brain regions are the prefrontal and cingulate cortices and the nucleus accumbens.
     (c)  False (p. 97): extrapyramidal side-effects emerge with greater than 80% receptor blockade. *In vivo* receptor occupancy of over 75% is found with therapeutic doses.
     (d)  True (p. 97): also true for $D_4:D_5$ ratio and $D_1:D_2$.
     (e)  False (p. 97): it is an agonist, and is used to suppress galactorrhoea and postpartum lactation.

30   Noradrenaline:
(a)   Noradrenaline neurones originate in the brain-stem.
(b)   Noradrenaline does not cross the blood–brain barrier.
(c)   Presynaptic alpha$_2$ adrenoceptors are involved in the control of noradrenaline release.
(d)   A significant loss of noradrenergic neurons is found in Parkinson's disease.
(e)   Clonidine is a noradrenaline antagonist.

31   Serotonin (5-HT):
(a)   The supply of L-tryptophan is the rate-limiting step in the synthesis of 5-HT.
(b)   Low levels of 5-HT have been shown to relate to violent or impulsive behaviour.
(c)   5-HT$_{1A}$ receptors are concentrated in the choroid plexus.
(d)   LSD is a 5-HT$_4$ agonist.
(e)   Almost all of the 5-HT in the blood is stored in platelets.

32   Peptides:
(a)   Starvation leads to increased CSF levels of endorphin in anorexia nervosa.
(b)   There is an absent euphoric response to opioids in depression.
(c)   CSF levels of thyrotrophin-releasing hormone (TRH) are increased in depression.
(d)   TRH reverses sedation of alcohol.
(e)   Injections of corticotrophin-releasing hormone (CRH) reduce appetite.

33   Frontal cerebral damage may be supported by the presence of the following:
(a)   Palmo-mental reflex.
(b)   Pout reflex.
(c)   Grasp reflex.
(d)   Groping reflex.
(e)   Counter-pull response.

34   Dominant parietal lobe lesions are indicated by:
(a)   Paraphasic fluent speech.
(b)   Anomia.
(c)   Impaired reading and writing.
(d)   Non-fluent aphasia with intact comprehension.
(e)   Ideomotor dyspraxia.

30　(a)　True (p. 98): from a series of nuclei, including the locus coeruleus.
　　(b)　True (p. 99): nor its metabolites with the exception of MHPG.
　　(c)　True (p. 101).
　　(d)　True (p. 102): also in Alzheimer's and Korsakoff's dementia.
　　(e)　False (p. 102): clonidine is a noradrenergic agonist.

31　(a)　True (p. 103).
　　(b)　False (p. 104): low levels of 5-HIAA have been shown to relate to or predict violent or impulsive behaviour, including murder, arson and self-harm.
　　(c)　False (p. 105): in several brain-stem nuclei, especially the dorsal and median Raphe cell bodies/hippocampus.
　　(d)　False (p. 105): it is a $5\text{-HT}_{2A}$ and $5\text{-HT}_{2B}$ agonist.
　　(e)　True (p. 104).

32　(a)　True (p. 108): this may explain the addiction to weight loss.
　　(b)　True (p. 108): this may indicate that an abnormality of mu receptors underlies anhedonia in this condition.
　　(c)　True (p. 110).
　　(d)　True (p. 110).
　　(e)　True (p. 109): also reduce sex drive.

33　(a)　True (p. 116): this is the most sensitive frontal release sign. It may be produced by firmly drawing a key across the thenar eminence of the hand while observing the mentalis area below the mouth. Contraction of the mentalis on the same side indicates frontal cerebral cortical damage or degeneration on the opposite side.
　　(b)　True (p. 117): tapping the lips with a vertically held pen may evoke this.
　　(c)　True (p. 117).
　　(d)　True (p. 117).
　　(e)　True (p. 117): *Gegenhalten*, when the patient actively resists attempts to passively flex or extend limb joint, is an indication of diffuse damage.

34　(a)　True (p. 120).
　　(b)　True (p. 120): this is an inability to name objects, usually on the left.
　　(c)　True (p. 120).
　　(d)　False (p. 120): left lateral frontal lesion.
　　(e)　False (p. 120): parietal dominant lobe lesion. Ideomotor praxis, the impairment of ability to perform motor tasks on verbal command, can be tested by asking the patient to salute, shrug the shoulders, etc.

Note. Additionally, dyscalculia (impairment of ability to perform simple calculations), finger agnosia, right/left disorientation and dysgraphia (Gerstmann's syndrome) indicate a dominant parietal lobe lesion. Non-dominant parietal lesions may produce spatial neglect, constructional dyspraxia, dressing dyspraxia.

35   Gerstmann's syndrome has the following features:

(a)   Right–left orientation.
(b)   Finger agnosia.
(c)   Dysgraphia.
(d)   Dyscalculia.
(e)   Constructional dyspraxia.


36   Primary generalised absence seizures:

(a)   Over 90% cease by late adolescence.
(b)   Most attacks last less than 1 minute.
(c)   They are associated with swallowing.
(d)   Diagnosis confirmed by hypsarrhythmia on EEG.
(e)   They are not easily triggered by hyperventilation.


37   Blepharospasm:

(a)   Blepharospasm is a dystonia.
(b)   Most cases are in association with Parkinsonism.
(c)   There is an association with brain-stem infarction.
(d)   Onset is usually in the third decade.
(e)   There is an association with nasal decongestants.


38   Tardive dyskinesia:

(a)   Tardive dyskinesia is characterised by athetoid movements of face and mouth.
(b)   It less frequently involves limbs and trunk.
(c)   It is commoner in patients receiving intermittent anticholinergic therapy.
(d)   The overall prevalence for people receiving long-term neuroleptic therapy is 40%.
(e)   Use of a more potent dopamine-blocking drug aggravates the condition in the short term.


39   Kleine–Levin syndrome:

(a)   The syndrome affects females predominantly.
(b)   Sufferers are usually under the age of 25 years.
(c)   Patient sleeps for 20 hours or more per day during an episode.
(d)   Hypersexuality is a feature.
(e)   Episodes last several days.


40   Parkinson's disease:

(a)   Parkinson's disease is a familial disorder with autosomal dominant transmission.
(b)   Mean age of onset is 65 years.
(c)   Severe disability or death occurs in about 40% of sufferers after 5 years.
(d)   It is characterised by a unilateral tremor typically at a frequency of 10 Hz.
(e)   Parkinsonism developing after the age of 60 years is generally considered to be atherosclerotic in origin.

35   (a)  False (p. 120): disorientation.
     (b)  True  (p. 120).
     (c)  True  (p. 120).
     (d)  True  (p. 120).
     (e)  False (p. 120): this is an impairment of visual spatial ability and indicates a non-dominant (usually parietal) lesion.

36   (a)  True  (p. 127): occurs predominantly in the early years.
     (b)  True  (p. 127): 30–45 seconds.
     (c)  True  (p. 128): also lip smacking and blinking.
     (d)  False (p. 128): 3 seconds per spike and wave.
     (e)  False (p. 128).

37   (a)  True  (p. 131): it is an adult-onset dystonia involving spasm of the orbicularis oculi and its associated muscles, leading to forced eye closure.
     (b)  False (p. 131): most cases are idiopathic, although it has been described in association with Parkinsonism, demyelinating disease and brain-stem infarction. It has also been induced by a variety of drugs.
     (c)  True  (p. 131).
     (d)  False (p. 131): fifth to sixth decade.
     (e)  True  (p. 131): has been associated with nasal decongestants, neuroleptics and levo-dopa.

38   (a)  True  (p. 132): or choreiform movements. In 80% of those affected, the dyskinesia is confined to the face and mouth, usually comprising tongue protrusion, lip smacking/pursing or grimacing.
     (b)  True  (p. 132).
     (c)  False (p. 132): concurrent anticholinergic therapy.
     (d)  False (p. 132): 25%.
     (e)  False (p. 132): produces short-term improvement, as does increasing the dose of neuroleptic. Reduction of dosage or withdrawal of neuroleptics causes an increase in severity in the short term, but in about 50% improvement or complete resolution follows.

39   (a)  False (p. 136): commoner in males.
     (b)  True  (p. 136).
     (c)  True  (p. 136).
     (d)  False (p. 137): hyperphagia, hypersomnia.
     (e)  True  (p. 136).

40   (a)  True  (p. 146): develops in about 25% of carriers.
     (b)  False (p. 146): 55 years.
     (c)  False (pp. 146–147): 25%.
     (d)  False (p. 147): 5 Hz and can be bilateral.
     (e)  True  (p. 147): presumed to be caused by infarction within the basal ganglia.

41 Features of Huntington's disease include:
(a) Autosomal dominant transmission with complete penetrance.
(b) Initial presentation often psychiatric.
(c) Subcortical dementia.
(d) Caudate tail atrophy.
(e) Profound weight loss.

42 The Trail Making Test assesses the following:
(a) Visual scanning.
(b) Number and letter sequencing.
(c) Rote memory.
(d) Visuomotor coordination.
(e) Psychomotor speed.

43 Tests of frontal lobe function include:
(a) Benton Verbal Fluency Test.
(b) Benton Visual Retention Test.
(c) Complex Figure of Rey.
(d) Speech Sound Perception Test.
(e) Halstead Category Test.

44 Tests of temporal lobe function include:
(a) Seashore Rhythms Test.
(b) Revised Wechsler Memory Scale.
(c) Left–Right Disorientation Test.
(d) Block Design.
(e) Object Assembly.

45 Studies on populations with schizophrenia and presenting with predominantly negative symptoms indicate:
(a) A significant higher ventricle:brain ratio.
(b) An overall deterioration in IQ.
(c) Short-term memory disturbances.
(d) Deficits in higher-order reasoning.
(e) Perceptual difficulties.

41  (a)  True (p. 147).
    (b)  True (p. 147): usually personality change, affective or schizophreni-
         form disorders, usually in the third or fourth decade, although earlier
         onset and later onset can occur.
    (c)  True (p. 147): blunting of drive and a global impairment of cognition.
    (d)  False (p. 147): the head of the caudate is characteristically, though
         not invariably, atrophied.
    (e)  True (p. 147): continuous movements may lead to profound weight
         loss.

42  (a)  True (p. 156).
    (b)  True (p. 156).
    (c)  True (p. 156).
    (d)  True (p. 156).
    (e)  True (p. 156).

43  (a)  True (p. 157).
    (b)  False (p. 157): it is a test of temporal lobe function.
    (c)  False (p. 157): it is a test of temporal lobe and parietal lobe function.
    (d)  False (p. 157): it is a test of temporal lobe function.
    (e)  True (p. 157).

         Note. Other frontal lobe tests include the Trail Making Test and the Wisconsin
         Card-Sorting Test.

44  (a)  True (p. 157).
    (b)  True (p. 157).
    (c)  False (p. 157): it is a test of parietal lobe function.
    (d)  False (p. 157): it is a test of parietal lobe function.
    (e)  False (p. 157): it is a test of parietal lobe function.

         Note. Other temporal lobe tests include the Speech Sound Perception Test and
         the Complex Figure of Rey.

45  (a)  True (p. 160).
    (b)  True (p. 160).
    (c)  True (p. 160).
    (d)  True (p. 160).
    (e)  True (p. 160).

46  Patients with schizophrenia tend to perform poorly on the following neuropsychological tests:
(a)  Wisconsin Card-Sort Test.
(b)  Speech Sounds Perception Test.
(c)  Trails A of the Halstead–Reitan Battery.
(d)  Weakening of dominance of the left hand in comparison with the right.
(e)  Category Test.

47  Retrograde amnesia:
(a)  Refers to memory impairment immediately before injury.
(b)  Is an unreliable index of injury prognosis.
(c)  Is an unreliable index of injury severity.
(d)  Constitutes a disturbance of memory for personal events and experiences.
(e)  Is considered to arise directly from shear forces within the brain.

48  Duration of post-traumatic amnesia is a good predictor of:
(a)  Recovery.
(b)  Long-term neurological outcome.
(c)  Long-term psychiatric outcome.
(d)  Occupational outcome.
(e)  Severity of cognitive disturbance.

49  Wechsler Adult Intelligence Scale – Revised:
(a)  Comprises eight sub-scales.
(b)  Assesses auditory concentration.
(c)  Assesses constructional ability.
(d)  Assesses visual–verbal integration.
(e)  Tests an attempt to draw a complex design from memory.

46  (a)  True (p. 161).
    (b)  True (p. 161).
    (c)  False (p. 161): Trails B of the Halstead–Reitan Battery, which specifically assesses the ability to shift flexibility between cognitive sets, inflexibility being most clearly associated with frontal lobe function.
    (d)  False (p. 161): weakening of dominance of the right hand in comparison with the left, as manifested by reduced finger tapping speed.
    (e)  True (p. 161): on tests such as the Category Test and Wisconsin Card-Sorting Test (which assess higher-order reasoning), people with schizophrenia do far more poorly than controls or other psychiatric controls.

    Note. There is a tendency for people with schizophrenia to perform poorly on tests that assess frontal and temporal function. In addition there is evidence to indicate specific disturbances of short-term memory, especially verbal short-term memory.

47  (a)  True (p. 165).
    (b)  True (p. 166).
    (c)  True (p. 166): extended periods of retrograde amnesia can occur in head-injury victims who suffer neither loss of consiousness nor impairment.
    (d)  True (p. 166): prior general information and knowledge may be only partially impaired and skilled behaviour unaffected.
    (e)  True (p. 165): and rotational movement of the brain within the skull.

    Note. The duration normally shrinks as the patient recovers. It also is characterised by islands of memory.

48  (a)  True (p. 167).
    (b)  True (p. 167).
    (c)  True (p. 167).
    (d)  True (p. 167).
    (e)  True (p. 166).

49  (a)  False (p. 178): 11 sub-scales.
    (b)  True (p. 178).
    (c)  True (p. 178).
    (d)  True (p. 178).
    (e)  False (p. 179): Rey–Osteirreith Figure is a test of immediate and delayed recall of complex spatial material. Also assesses planning and constructional ability. The subject first copies a complex design, then attempts to draw it from memory.

50   The following are tests of information processing:
(a)   Stroop Colour–Word Interference Test.
(b)   Trail Making Test.
(c)   Visual Search Test.
(d)   Benton Verbal Fluency Test.
(e)   Revised Token Test.


51   Neuropsychological tests which assess language function include:
(a)   Revised Token Test.
(b)   Boston Diagnostic Aphasia Examination.
(c)   Rey Auditory Verbal Learning Test.
(d)   Adult Memory and Information Processing Battery.
(e)   Dichotic Listening Test.


52   Macroscopic findings in Alzheimer's disease include:
(a)   Plaques.
(b)   Pallor of locus coeruleus.
(c)   Reduction in brain weight.
(d)   Enlargement of the lateral and third ventricles.
(e)   Narrowing of sulci in a fronto-tempero-parietal distribution.

50 (a) True (p. 180): assesses speed of processing for simple verbal and non-verbal information. Also assesses cognitive ability. Comprises three components: reading out rapidly an array of 100 words made up of random presentations of the words RED, GREEN, BLUE; reading out the colour hues RED, GREEN and BLUE; the words RED, GREEN and BLUE are written in coloured ink such that the colour hue does not match the colour word. Subjects read out the colour hue only.

   (b) True (p. 180): measures visual scanning, visuomotor coordination, psychomotor ability, sequencing, category alternation.

   (c) True (p. 180): assesses pattern recognition, visual scanning, speed of visuospatial processing. Subjects pick out a pattern from an array which correctly matches a central pattern.

   (d) False (p. 180): language function – assesses fluency and word-finding ability. Subjects are required to say as many words as they can beginning with specific letters of the alphabet in 1 minute.

   (e) False (p. 180): language function (receptive language skills). The use of a motor response makes this a useful tool with individuals with expressive language difficulties.

   Note. One additional test is the Paced Auditory Serial Addition Test, which assesses attentional processes, monitoring, tracking and sequencing, and speed of computational processing. Subjects listen to a series of numbers presented at defined time intervals and have to add up successive pairs.

51 (a) True (p. 180): assesses receptive language skills. The use of a motor response makes this a useful tool with individuals with expressive language difficulties.

   (b) True (p. 179): assesses a wide range of receptive and expressive language.

   (c) False (p. 179): memory function.

   (d) False (p. 179): memory function.

   (e) False (p. 181): test of laterality.

52 (a) False (p. 198): microscopic finding, as are tangles, though both are non-specific.

   (b) True (p. 198).

   (c) True (p. 198): in comparison with normal age-matched controls.

   (d) True (p. 198).

   (e) False (p. 198): widening of sulci.

53   Neurofibrillary tangles have the following properties:
(a)   They are especially found in Ammon's horn.
(b)   They are found in the same sites as senile plaques.
(c)   Extracellular amyloid is a component.
(d)   Beta A4 protein is a major biochemical component.
(e)   Abnormally phosphorylated tau protein is present in tangles.

54   Neurofibrillary tangles occur:
(a)   With ageing.
(b)   In Down's syndrome.
(c)   In dementia pugilistica.
(d)   In postencephalitic Parkinson's disease.
(e)   In progressive supranuclear palsy.

55   Neuropathological features of Pick's disease include:
(a)   Knife-edge gyri.
(b)   Temporal atrophy.
(c)   Pick bodies, which are round, argyrophilic intraneuronal inclusions.
(d)   Pick cells, which are swollen cortical pyramidal cells.
(e)   Nerve cell loss.

56   In relation to the neuropathology of Huntington's disease the following
      are correct:
(a)   There is striatal atrophy.
(b)   There is flattening of the outline of the head of the caudate.
(c)   Gliosis can be marked.
(d)   There is cortical atrophy.
(e)   There are no specific microscopic abnormalities.

57   Neuropathological findings in Creutzfeldt–Jakob disease include:
(a)   Plaques are rarely present.
(b)   There is nerve cell loss.
(c)   There is gliosis.
(d)   Spongiform change.
(e)   There may be no macroscopic abnormalities.

58   Neuropathological features of Parkinson's disease include:
(a)   Pallor of substantia nigra.
(b)   Pallor of locus coeruleus.
(c)   Lewy bodies in the nucleus of Meynert.
(d)   Nerve cell loss.
(e)   Intraneuronal inclusions in the sympathetic nuclei.

53  (a)  True (p. 199): especially in the hippocampus. Also found in the
         amygdala, parahippocampal gyrus, neocortex, locus coeruleus,
         nucleus of Meynert, Raphe nuclei.
    (b)  True (p. 199).
    (c)  False (p. 199): plaques include extracellular amyloid as a component.
    (d)  False (p. 199): beta A4 protein is a major biochemical component
         of plaque amyloid.
    (e)  True (p. 199): in the parahippocampal gyrus.

         Note. Tangles form within nerve cell bodies, particularly in the pyramidal cells
         of the hippocampus, where they are flame-shaped. They are composed of
         paired helical filaments.

54  (a)  True (p. 199).
    (b)  True (p. 199).
    (c)  True (p. 199).
    (d)  True (p. 199).
    (e)  True (p. 199).

55  (a)  True (p. 200): in the context of dramatic frontal or temporal atrophy.
    (b)  True (p. 200).
    (c)  True (p. 200): microscopic finding.
    (d)  True (p. 200): microscopic finding.
    (e)  True (p. 200).

56  (a)  True (p. 200).
    (b)  True (p. 200): or even concavity.
    (c)  True (p. 200).
    (d)  True (p. 200).
    (e)  True (p. 200): although the large striatal neurons are relatively well
         preserved in comparison with the small and medium-sized ones.

57  (a)  True (p. 200): without obvious abnormal neurites.
    (b)  True (p. 200).
    (c)  True (p. 200).
    (d)  True (p. 200).
    (e)  True (p. 200): or the brain may appear atrophic.

58  (a)  True (p. 201).
    (b)  True (p. 201).
    (c)  True (p. 201): also in substantia nigra and locus coeruleus.
    (d)  True (p. 201): usually in areas where the inclusions are seen.
    (e)  True (p. 201): these are Lewy bodies (eosinophilic and haloed).

59 Nicotinic acid deficiency leads to:

(a) Pellagra.
(b) White matter degeneration in spinal cord.
(c) Mania.
(d) Paranoid states.
(e) Ophthalmoplegia of lateral gaze.

60 Neuropathological findings in schizophrenia include:

(a) Lateral ventricles are abnormally large, especially in the temporal lobe.
(b) Brain weight is normal.
(c) Brain size is reduced.
(d) The anterior parahippocampal gyrus is particularly severely affected.
(e) Right side is probably more involved than left.

61 The paraventricular nucleus (PVN):

(a) Neurons synthesising oxytocin connect the PVN with the posterior pituitary.
(b) TRH is synthesised in the PVN.
(c) CRF is synthesised in the PVN.
(d) Neurons within the PVN affect peripheral thermogenesis.
(e) The PVN is situated in the thalamus.

62 Stimuli for release of posterior pituitary hormones (oxytocin and arginine vasopressin, AVP) include:

(a) Increased plasma osmolality.
(b) Nausea.
(c) Labour.
(d) Stress.
(e) Atrial peptides.

63 In relation to growth hormone the following statements are true:

(a) It regulates lipid metabolism.
(b) There is a nocturnal surge during fast-wave sleep.
(c) Stimulated serum growth hormone levels are generally lower in pre-menopausal than postmenopausal women.
(d) Its release is inhibited by somatostatin.
(e) Growth hormone inhibits peripheral production of the insulin-like growth factor IGF-I.

59 (a) True (p. 210).
   (b) False (p. 210): $B_{12}$ deficiency results in white matter degeneration in spinal cord.
   (c) True (p. 210): also depression.
   (d) True (p. 210).
   (e) False (p. 209): thymine deficiency leads to ophthalmoplegia of lateral gaze.

60 (a) True (p. 212): where there appears to be less grey matter than normal.
   (b) False (p. 212): brain weight and size are decreased.
   (c) True (p. 212).
   (d) True (p. 212): also the hippocampus.
   (e) False (p. 212): left side is probably more involved than the right side.

   Note. The degree of these changes relates more closely to negative than to positive symptoms.

61 (a) True (p. 235): also true for ADH.
   (b) True (p. 235).
   (c) True (p. 235): and transported to the median eminence and released into the hypothalamopituitary portal circulation to stimulate hormone release by ACTH-releasing cells.
   (d) True (p. 235): also affect feeding, gastrointestinal function and cardio-vascular function, transported to the median eminence and released into the hypothalamopituitary portal circulation to stimulate hormone release by TSH-releasing cells.
   (e) False (p. 235): it is situated in the hypothalamus and is a site for the reception of afferent signals from the brain-stem, higher cerebral centres and other hypothalamic nuclei.

62 (a) False (p. 238): decreased plasma osmolality leads to release of AVP.
   (b) True (p. 238): AVP.
   (c) True (p. 238): oxytocin, which is also released by the suckling reflex.
   (d) True (p. 238): AVP.
   (e) True (p. 238): AVP.

63 (a) True (p. 239): also true for carbohydrate metabolism.
   (b) False (p. 240): there is a nocturnal surge during slow-wave stage 3–4 sleep.
   (c) False (p. 240): stimulated serum growth hormone levels are generally higher in premenopausal than postmenopausal women.
   (d) True (p. 240).
   (e) False (p. 239): it stimulates it.

64  The following are true statements with reference to the control of growth hormone release:

(a)  Somatostatin has an indirect inhibitory influence on the production of growth hormone.
(b)  Somatostatin exerts a tonic inhibitory influence on growth hormone.
(c)  Muscarinic cholinergic agonists inhibit basal growth hormone release.
(d)  Hypothyroidism causes a profound suppression of growth hormone production in the pituitary.
(e)  Corticosteroids increase growth hormone production and release.

65  The normal EEG:

(a)  Delta waves have a frequency below 3.5 Hz.
(b)  The voltage of the scalp-recorded EEG activity in adults is usually between 300 and 500 $\mu$V.
(c)  The frequency of the dominant occipital alpha activity tends to increase in the elderly.
(d)  Alpha activity is temporarily blocked by eye opening.
(e)  Theta and delta activity is normal in the young.

66  Treatment effects on the EEG:

(a)  Therapeutic effects of barbiturates produce excess fast activity and slow activity.
(b)  Withdrawal of hypnotic drugs after long-term use may produce paroxysmal complex spike activity.
(c)  Phenothiazines produce minor increase in alpha frequencies at therapeutic levels.
(d)  Benzodiazepines are not associated with changes in fast frequencies.
(e)  Anti-epileptic drugs cause increased slow-wave activity.

67  The following EEG diagnostic features are correct:

(a)  Herpes simplex encephalitis causes episodic discharges recurring every 1–3 seconds.
(b)  A non-specific increase in slow waves occurs diffusely over the scalp in neurosyphilis.
(c)  Periodic stereotyped repetitive discharges in the EEG at a rate of 1 per second are strongly suggestive of subacute sclerosing panencephalitis.
(d)  An EEG showing high-amplitude repetitive bilaterally synchronous symmetrical polyphasic sharp-wave and slow-wave complexes at a rate of one every 10 seconds is characteristic of Creutzfeldt–Jakob disease.
(e)  There are no specific abnormalities on EEG in meningitis.

64 (a) False (p. 241): somatostatin has a direct inhibitory influence on the production of growth hormone.
   (b) True (p. 241).
   (c) False (p. 241): stimulate basal growth hormone release.
   (d) True (p. 242).
   (e) True (p. 242).

65 (a) True (p. 247): usually 0.1–3.5 Hz (theta 4–7.5 Hz, alpha 8–13 Hz, beta above 13 Hz, usually 14–40 Hz).
   (b) False (p. 248): usually between 10 and 100 µV.
   (c) False (p. 248): the frequency of the dominant occipital alpha activity tends to slow in the elderly, apparently reflecting underlying cerebral pathology, either vascular or degenerative.
   (d) True (pp. 248–249): as well as a variety of alerting stimuli.
   (e) True (p. 249): theta and delta activity is normal in the young and during sleep.

66 (a) True (p. 255): and EEG changes characteristic of drowsiness and sleep. Changes are usually most prominent in the first few days.
   (b) True (p. 255): especially on photic stimulation.
   (c) True (p. 255): also produce slow-wave paroxysmal complex activity at higher doses.
   (d) False (p. 255): benzodiazepines produce a significant increase in fast activity which persists for up to 2 weeks after the drug has been stopped.
   (e) True (p. 255): carbamazepine is related to the tricyclic antidepressants and can give rise to slow and paroxysmal complex disturbances.

67 (a) True (p. 257): also variable focal slow waves over the temporal areas.
   (b) True (p. 257): also true for several parasitic infestations and Reye's syndrome.
   (c) False (p. 259): high-amplitude repetitive, bilaterally synchronous and symmetrical, polyphasic sharp-wave and slow-wave complexes which occur every 4–15 seconds are characteristic of the condition.
   (d) False (p. 258): periodic stereotyped repetitive discharges in the EEG at a rate of about 1 per second, although not invariably present, particularly in the early stages of the disease, are strongly suggestive of the diagnosis.
   (e) True (p. 257): the degree of EEG slowing is dependent on the extent to which the cerebral hemispheres are involved.

68 EEG indicators of good outcome following head injury include:

(a) The presence of spindles in the acute stage.
(b) Reactivity with alerting response stimuli.
(c) In prolonged coma states the re-emergence of circadian rhythms.
(d) An increase in frequency of slow activity for recovery from the 'apallic' state.
(e) The presence of sleep patterns in prolonged coma.

69 EEG findings in absence seizures include:

(a) Regular 3 Hz complexes.
(b) May include multiple spike- and slow-wave complexes.
(c) Bilateral abnormalities.
(d) The EEG inter-ictal expression of background activity is usually normal.
(e) Symmetrical activity.

70 Sleep and EEG:

(a) Alpha spindles occur in stage 1.
(b) K complexes occur in stages 2, 3 and 4.
(c) REM is characterised by desynchronisation with faster frequencies.
(d) Stage 4 is characterised by sleep spindles of fast activity.
(e) Frequent vertex sharp waves occur in stage 4.

71 Evoked potentials:

(a) Visual evoked potential (VEP) abnormalities are pathologically specific.
(b) The pattern VEP is independent of visual acuity.
(c) High-amplitude evoked potentials are seen in myoclonic epilepsy.
(d) Brain-stem auditory evoked potentials arise from subcortical structures.
(e) Somatosensory evoked potentials depend on the integrity of the distal sensory afferent nerves.

68  (a) True  (p. 263): increase in frequency of slow activity also. It indicates intact cortical function.
    (b) True  (p. 263).
    (c) True  (p. 263): also re-emergence of sleep patterns.
    (d) True  (p. 264): also the reappearance of alpha waves. The 'apallic' state is characterised clinically by an awake but unaware condition, following prolonged coma.
    (e) True  (p. 263).

69  (a) True  (p. 269).
    (b) True  (p. 269).
    (c) True  (p. 269).
    (d) True  (p. 269).
    (e) True  (p. 269).

70  (a) True  (p. 283).
    (b) True  (p. 283).
    (c) True  (p. 283).
    (d) False  (p. 283): stage 3 is characterised by marked slow activity, K complexes and some spindles.
    (e) False  (p. 283): vertex sharp waves occur in stage 2.

71  (a) False  (p. 294).
    (b) False  (pp. 294–295): very sensitive to a reduction of visual acuity.
    (c) True  (p. 295).
    (d) True  (p. 296).
    (e) True  (p. 297).

    Note. Evoked potentials reveal neuronal reponses to sensory stimuli and are directly related to the functional integrity of neurological pathways.

# Psychology and the Social Sciences

1   In relation to Piaget's stages of cognitive development the following
    are true of the sensorimotor stage:
(a)   It spans from birth to 3 years.
(b)   The child can distinguish self and non-self.
(c)   The child is egocentric.
(d)   Perception is subordinate to action.
(e)   There is difficulty concerning objects not present.

2   The following statements regarding Piaget's stages of cognitive
    development are true:
(a)   Preoperational stage lasts approximately 5 years.
(b)   Failure to recognise conservation of different quantities is a feature of the
      preoperational stage.
(c)   Logical reasoning is not present until formal operational stage.
(d)   Non-logical thought is a feature of ages 2–7 years.
(e)   A child's failure to make transitive inferences is a feature of the concrete
      operational stage.

3   According to Seligman the following parallels between helplessness
    and depression exist:
(a)   Both result in lowered levels of voluntary behaviour.
(b)   Both produce a negative cognitive set.
(c)   Both have a similar time course of persistence.
(d)   Both produce increased levels of aggression.
(e)   Both produce cholinergic underactivation.

4   The following therapies are extinction procedures:
(a)   Massed learning.
(b)   Flooding.
(c)   Implosion therapy.
(d)   Systematic desensitisation.
(e)   Contingency learning.

5   Speech in Broca's aphasia has the following features:
(a)   Rapid.
(b)   Fluent.
(c)   Largely preserved syntax.
(d)   Marked impairments in semantic comprehension.
(e)   Marked impairment in correct use of content words.

225

1  (a)  False (p. 4): from birth to 2 years.
   (b)  False (p. 4): this relates to the preoperational stage.
   (c)  False (p. 4): this relates to the preoperational stage.
   (d)  True (p. 4).
   (e)  True (p. 4).

2  (a)  True (p. 4).
   (b)  True (p. 5): but they have some understanding of conservation.
   (c)  False (p. 5): logical reasoning is not present until ages 7–12 years, that is, the concrete operational stage.
   (d)  True (p. 4).
   (e)  False (p. 6): this relates to the preoperational stage.

3  (a)  True (p. 27).
   (b)  True (p. 27).
   (c)  True (p. 27).
   (d)  False (p. 27): both produce decreased levels of aggression.
   (e)  False (p. 27): both produce cholinergic overactivation and noradrenergic depletion; both also decrease appetite.

4  (a)  True (p. 29): this is sustained and repeated exposure to a phobic object.
   (b)  True (p. 29): this is exposure to phobic objects.
   (c)  True (p. 29).
   (d)  True (p. 29).
   (e)  False (p. 27).

5  (a)  False (p. 92).
   (b)  False (p. 92).
   (c)  False (p. 92).
   (d)  False (p. 92).
   (e)  False (p. 92).
       Note. All of these are true for Wernicke's aphasia.

6    Wernicke's aphasia may have the following speech features:
(a)  Agrammatism.
(b)  Profound lack of syntactic structure.
(c)  Words are produced one at a time.
(d)  Word substitution.
(e)  Paraphasias.

7    The performance scale of the Wechsler Adult Intelligence Scale – Revised (WAIS–R) includes:
(a)  Block completion.
(b)  Picture design.
(c)  Digit symbol.
(d)  Similarities.
(e)  Arithmetic.

8    The following statements are true with regard to the Wechsler Memory Scale – Revised:
(a)  Broadly assesses long-term memory.
(b)  Takes less than 1 hour to administer.
(c)  Tests figural memory.
(d)  Tests visual reproduction.
(e)  Tests paired associate learning.

9    Components of the Halstead–Reitan Neuropsychological Battery (HRNB) include:
(a)  Minnesota Multiphasic Personality Inventory.
(b)  Category Test.
(c)  Dynanometer.
(d)  Paired associate learning.
(e)  Stroop Colour–Word Interference Test.

10   The following are correct statements:
(a)  By age 2 months an infant will recognise a caregiver.
(b)  Fear of strange children does not occur until the second year of life.
(c)  Fear of adult strangers occurs at the end of the first year.
(d)  The primary attachment figure will be the person who provides most care to the child.
(e)  The child's first attachment relationship should be formed in the first year of life to ensure subsequent socio-emotional well-being.

6   (a) False (p. 92): this is true for Broca's aphasia.
    (b) False (p. 92): this is true for Broca's aphasia.
    (c) False (p. 92): this is true for Broca's aphasia.
    (d) True (p. 92).
    (e) True (p. 92).

   Note. Word substitution and paraphasias in extreme cases is known as jargon aphasia. Speech is replete and sometimes neologisms occur.

7   (a) False (p. 116): block design and block assembly are features of the performance scale of the WAIS-R.
    (b) False (p. 116): picture completion and picture arrangement are features of the performance scale of the WAIS-R.
    (c) True (p. 116).
    (d) False (p. 116): this is part of the verbal scale.
    (e) False (p. 116): this is part of the verbal scale.

8   (a) False (p. 116): short-term memory and learning are broadly assessed.
    (b) True (p. 116).
    (c) True (p. 117): visual recognition memory.
    (d) True (p. 117).
    (e) True (p. 117): it tests new verbal learning ability.

9   (a) True (p. 117).
    (b) True (p. 117): assesses hypothesis formation and testing, planning and organisation.
    (c) True (p. 117): assesses dominant and non-dominant hand grip strength.
    (d) False (p. 117): this is a feature of the Wechsler Memory Scale.
    (e) False (p. 118).

   Note. The HRNB is used to diagnose brain damage and has 11 components: Wechsler Adult Intelligence Scale; Minnesota Multiphasic Personality Inventory; Trail Making Test; Category Test; Speech Sounds Perception Test; Seashore Rhythm Test; Aphasia Screen; Tactual Performance Test; Finger Oscillation Test; Dynanometer; Sensory Perceptual Examination.

10  (a) False (p. 156): occurs somewhere between 7 and 8 months (though the exact age is contentious). The child should also show distress at his or her departure.
    (b) True (p. 157).
    (c) True (p. 157).
    (d) False (p. 158).
    (e) False (p. 158).

11 Factors found to be important in predicting high relapse rates in patients diagnosed with schizophrenia include:
(a) Critical comments.
(b) Hostility.
(c) Emotional over-involvement.
(d) Levels of expressed emotion greater than 35 hours per week in the home.
(e) Low level of face-to-face contact and communication.

12 Parsons' discussion of the 'sick role' notes the following features:
(a) Exemption from normal social role responsibilities.
(b) The exemption above is not automatic.
(c) The ill person is 'under an obligation to want to get well'.
(d) The ill person has an obligation to consult a doctor.
(e) Ill people are in a condition that must be 'taken care of'.

13 With reference to the sociology of illness the following are true:
(a) Illness and death rates show a curvilinear relationship with age.
(b) In industrial societies men tend to live as long as women.
(c) In industrial societies women report more ill health.
(d) Premature death is more common among those of lower social class.
(e) African–Caribbean psychiatric residents in Western societies tend to have a higher mortality rate.

11  (a)  True  (p. 251).
    (b)  True  (p. 251).
    (c)  True  (p. 251).
    (d)  True  (p. 252).
    (e)  False  (p. 252): this is a protective factor.

12  (a)  True  (p. 319).
    (b)  True  (p. 319): illness has to be legitimised.
    (c)  True  (p. 320).
    (d)  True  (p. 320): that is, an obligation to seek technically competent help.
    (e)  True  (p. 319).

13  (a)  True  (pp. 322–323): high rates in infancy with a decline in children and then a further increase in rate with middle age and old age.
    (b)  False  (p. 323): women live longer.
    (c)  True  (p. 323): they also make more use of health services.
    (d)  True  (p. 323).
    (e)  True  (p. 323): also true for morbidity rate and also in prison inmates.

# Old Age Psychiatry

1   The following are true of the cognitive rating scales:
(a)   The Abbreviated Mental State Score is almost entirely an orientation and concentration test.
(b)   The Mini-Mental State Examination has a cut-off score of 25/30.
(c)   The comprehensive Clifton Assessment Procedure for the Elderly (CAPE) has an information/orientation sub-scale.
(d)   The CAMCOG is a cognitive sub-scale of the Cambridge Examination for Mental Disorders of the Elderly (CAMDEX).
(e)   The Clock Drawing Test offers qualitative and quantitative information.

2   The Geriatric Depression Scale:
(a)   Is designed to avoid questions concerning somatic symptoms.
(b)   Was originally a 30-item test but now has 15 items.
(c)   Enables most subjects to be scored for depression in 4–5 minutes.
(d)   Suggests the possibility of depression if the overall score is 10 or more.
(e)   Consists of a series of statements in large print on cards to which the patient is required to respond 'true' or 'false'.

3   The CAMDEX incorporates:
(a)   Mini Mental State Examination.
(b)   Blessed Dementia Rating Scale (BDRS).
(c)   Hachinski Ischaemia Score.
(d)   CAMCOG.
(e)   Montgomery–Åsberg Depression Rating Scale.

4   ICD–10 criteria for delirium include:
(a)   Reduced ability to shift attention.
(b)   Visual hallucinations.
(c)   Delusions.
(d)   Hypoactivity.
(e)   Nightmares.

5   Delirium differs from dementia in the following ways:
(a)   It has a consistent course.
(b)   It features early/occasional lucid spells.
(c)   Sundowning always occurs.
(d)   There is usually normal alertness.
(e)   Orientation is more consistently impaired.

1　(a)　False (p. 10): it is an orientation and memory test. The cut-off score is 7/10 or 8/10 and it takes a few minutes to use.

　　(b)　False (p. 10): 24/30 is the cut-off. It takes 5–10 minutes to complete. It covers orientation, memory, concentration, language, praxis and agnosis.

　　(c)　True (p. 10): It has 12 questions.

　　(d)　True (p. 12): CAMCOG is a comprehensive cognitive test which covers a wide range of ability. It gives a score out of 104.

　　(e)　True (p. 10): it is a test of praxis.

2　(a)　True (p. 12): it is designed to avoid questions concerning somatic symptoms and function which in older patients might be accounted for by physical disorders, sleep disturbance or weight loss.

　　(b)　True (p. 13).

　　(c)　True (p. 13).

　　(d)　False (p. 13): an overall score of 5 or more suggests the possibility of depression.

　　(e)　False (p. 13): this is the Brief Assessment Schedule Depression Cards (BASDEC), which was initially designed for use in liaison psychiatry and is especially useful for deaf patients.

3　(a)　True (p. 14).

　　(b)　True (p. 14).

　　(c)　True (p. 14).

　　(d)　True (p. 14).

　　(e)　False (p. 13).

4　(a)　True (p. 29).

　　(b)　True (p. 29).

　　(c)　True (p. 29).

　　(d)　True (p. 29).

　　(e)　True (p. 29).

　　　　Note. Also true are impaired consciousness, perceptual disturbances, impairment of abstract thinking and comprehension, memory impairment, psychomotor disturbance, disorders of the sleep–wake cycle and emotional disturbance.

5　(a)　False (p. 39): it has a fluctuating course.

　　(b)　False (p. 39): lucid spells are common in delirium.

　　(c)　True (p. 39).

　　(d)　False (p. 39): usually heightened or reduced alertness.

　　(e)　False (p. 39): orientation is variably impaired.

6   Specific scales for assessment of delirium include:

(a)   Delirium Assessment Scale.
(b)   Delirium Confusional Interview.
(c)   Confusion Assessment Method Questionnaire.
(d)   Confusional State Evaluation.
(e)   Informant Questionnaire on Cognitive Decline in the Elderly.

7   Electroencephalogram (EEG) and delirium:

(a)   Is of frequent help in the diagnosis.
(b)   Typically shows slowing of delta rhythms.
(c)   Shows the emergence of alpha rhythms.
(d)   Shows bilaterally symmetrical predominant frontal waves.
(e)   Shows diffuse slowing in up to 80% of delirium patients.

8   Alzheimer's disease:

(a)   The prevalence rate is 3% in the age band 70–79 years.
(b)   Disorientation for place is more obvious than that for time.
(c)   Disorders of thought content occur in approximately 25% of patients.
(d)   Disorders of affect are relatively common.
(e)   Personality changes are a relatively late feature.

9   EEG in normal ageing shows:

(a)   A generalised slowing of alpha rhythm.
(b)   An increase in theta waves.
(c)   A decrease in delta activity.
(d)   A decrease in beta activity.
(e)   Paroxysmal sharp waves.

10   Factors associated with poorer survival in Alzheimer's disease include:

(a)   Frontal lobe damage.
(b)   Female gender.
(c)   Prominent behavioural abnormalities.
(d)   Apraxia.
(e)   Misidentification phenomenon.

6    (a)  False (p. 41): Delirium Rating Scale (DRS) has items which refer to aetiology and course. It was developed to complement DSM criteria.
     (b)  False (p. 41): Delirium Symptom Interview assesses three 'critical' symptoms – disorientation, disturbance of consciousness and perceptual disturbance – as well as disruption of the sleep–wake cycle, incoherence, altered psychomotor behaviour and fluctuations. It was designed to be usable by other than doctors.
     (c)  True  (p. 41): it is based on DSM–III criteria and requires the following for a diagnosis of delirium – acute changes in mental state, fluctuating course, inattention and either disorganised thinking or altered level of consciousness.
     (d)  True  (pp. 41–42): it has 12 core items – disorientation in four modes, thought, memory and concentration disturbances, distractibility, perseveration, impaired contact, paranoid ideation and hallucinations.
     (e)  True  (p. 42).

7    (a)  False (p. 42).
     (b)  False (p. 42): typically shows slowing of alpha rhythms.
     (c)  False (p. 42): shows the emergence of theta waves.
     (d)  True  (p. 42): shows bilaterally symmetrical predominant frontal delta waves.
     (e)  True  (p. 42).

8    (a)  True  (p. 51).
     (b)  False  (p. 51): disorientation for time is more obvious than that for place.
     (c)  False  (p. 52): disorders of thought content (delusions and paranoid ideation) occur in approximately 15% of patients.
     (d)  True  (p. 52): depression occurs in up to 50%, although it is usually mild.
     (e)  False  (p. 53): personality changes are a relatively early feature.

9    (a)  True  (p. 59).
     (b)  True  (p. 59).
     (c)  False (p. 59): an increase in delta activity.
     (d)  False (p. 59): an increase in beta activity.
     (e)  False (p. 54): paroxysmal sharp waves occur in Creutzfeld–Jacob disease with slow background rhythm.

     Note. Alzheimer's shows a normal tracing in early stages, followed by slowing of alpha and beta, with an increase in delta and theta waves.

10   (a)  False (p. 60): parietal lobe damage is associated with a poorer survival rate.
     (b)  False (p. 60): male gender.
     (c)  True  (p. 60): for example irritability and wandering.
     (d)  True  (p. 60).
     (e)  False (p. 60): the absence of misidentification phenomena despite its association with younger age.

     Note. Also age of onset of less than 65 years and depression observed by rater are factors associated with poorer survival in Alzheimer's disease.

11  In the genetics of Alzheimer's disease the following have been implicated:

(a)  Mutations have been found on chromosome 1 in the gene encoding for beta amyloid precursor.
(b)  Chromosome 14 is implicated in approximately 25% of cases of early-onset familial Alzheimer's disease.
(c)  The presenilin 1 gene has been identified on chromosome 1.
(d)  The gene cloned on chromosome 14 is presenilin 2.
(e)  The apolipoprotein E gene is situated on chromosome 19.

12  Neurofibrillary tangles occur in the following:

(a)  Progressive supranuclear palsy.
(b)  Pick's disease.
(c)  Amyotrophic lateral sclerosis.
(d)  Dementia pugilistica.
(e)  Lewy-body dementia.

13  The following occur in Pick's disease:

(a)  Neurofibrillary tangles.
(b)  Amyloid deposition.
(c)  Pick's bodies.
(d)  Hirano bodies.
(e)  Granulovacular degeneration.

14  Plaques have the following features:

(a)  Usually found in pyramidal cells of layers 3 and 4 of the cortex.
(b)  Spherical argyrophilic lesions.
(c)  Occur in senile dementia and old people.
(d)  Diagnostic significance of plaques is greater than that of tangles.
(e)  Neuropathological criteria for the diagnosis of Alzheimer's disease require more than 20 plaques in people between the ages of 66 and 75 years.

15  Neurotransmitter changes in Alzheimer's disease include:

(a)  Decreased dopamine beta-hydroxylase.
(b)  Increased dopamine.
(c)  Increased muscarinergic receptors.
(d)  Normal nicotinergic receptors.
(e)  Decreased somatostatin.

16  Binswanger's disease has the following features:

(a)  Progressive small-vessel disease.
(b)  Step-like intellectual decline.
(c)  Periventricular lucencies on brain imaging.
(d)  Subcortical dementia.
(e)  Commonly dysphasia as a specific deficit.

11  (a)  False (p. 61): chromosome 21.
    (b)  False (p. 61): chromosome 14 is implicated in approximately 75% of cases of early-onset Alzheimer's disease, whereas chromosome 21 is implicated in 25% of cases.
    (c)  False (p. 62): the presenilin 1 gene has been identified on chromosome 14.
    (d)  False (p. 62): the gene cloned on chromosome 1 is presenilin 2.
    (e)  True (p. 62).

12  (a)  True (p. 65).
    (b)  True (p. 65).
    (c)  True (p. 65).
    (d)  True (p. 65).
    (e)  True (p. 65).

    Note. Also true for ageing, Alzheimer's disease, Down's syndrome and Parkinson's disease.

13  (a)  True (p. 65).
    (b)  True (p. 65).
    (c)  True (p. 65).
    (d)  True (p. 65).
    (e)  True (p. 65).

14  (a)  False (p. 65): tangles are found in pyramidal cells of layers 3 and 4 of the cortex; plaques are found in the upper cortical layers.
    (b)  True (p. 65).
    (c)  True (p. 66).
    (d)  True (p. 66): because the number of plaques seems to be linked more closely with the degree of cognitive impairment.
    (e)  False (p. 66): more than 10 plaques per mm$^2$.

15  (a)  True (p. 69).
    (b)  False (p. 69): decrease in dopamine.
    (c)  False (p. 69): decrease in muscarinergic presynaptic M2 sub-class receptors.
    (d)  True (p. 69): no consistent change has been found.
    (e)  True (p. 69).

    Note. Also true are a decrease in choline-acetyltransferase, decreased acetylcholine, decreased noradrenaline, decreased serotonin, decreased GABA and decreased corticotrophin-releasing factor.

16  (a)  True (p. 75).
    (b)  True (p. 74): slow, gradual or step-like decline.
    (c)  True (p. 75): plus extensive white matter changes.
    (d)  True (p. 75).
    (e)  False (p. 75): this is more suggestive of cortical strokes.

17 The following are included within the Hachinski ischaemia score for vascular dementia:
(a) Depression.
(b) Somatic complaints.
(c) Emotional incontinence.
(d) Fluctuating course.
(e) Focal neurological signs.

18 Features of frontotemporal dementia include:
(a) Hyperorality.
(b) Preservation of insight.
(c) Fluent aphasia.
(d) Spatial disorientation.
(e) Behavioural problems.

19 Indications of depression in patients with dementia as featured in the Depressive Signs Scale include:
(a) Agitation.
(b) Slowness of movement.
(c) Slowness of speech.
(d) Alleviation of sad appearance by external circumstances.
(e) Hallucinations.

20 Depression in the elderly:
(a) The genetic contribution to depressive illness decreases with age.
(b) Depression in all age groups is more common in women.
(c) Depression in all age groups is associated with hypoactivity and dysregulation of the hypothalamic–pituitary–adrenal axis.
(d) The response of thyroid-stimulating hormone (TSH) to thyrotrophin- releasing hormone (TRH) is less age dependent than cortisol non-suppression.
(e) Variables measured during sleep show similar changes in depression and with ageing.

21 Late paraphrenia:
(a) Persecutory delusions are found in approximately 90% of patients.
(b) Auditory hallucinations are found in approximately 75%.
(c) Visual hallucinations are detected in up to 60%.
(d) First-rank symptoms are frequently seen.
(e) Tactile hallucinations are rare.

22 The following types of delusion are found in late paraphrenia:
(a) Control.
(b) Grandiosity.
(c) Gender.
(d) Religion.
(e) Misidentification.

17 (a) True (p. 76).
   (b) True (p. 76).
   (c) True (p. 76).
   (d) True (p. 76).
   (e) True (p. 76).

   Note. Also true are abrupt onset, step-wise deterioration, nocturnal confusion, relative preservation of personality, history of hypertension, history of strokes, atherosclerosis and focal neurological symptoms.

18 (a) True (p. 80).
   (b) False (p. 80): early loss of insight.
   (c) False (p. 80): non-fluent aphasia.
   (d) False (p. 80): spatial orientation is well preserved.
   (e) True (p. 80): personality changes.

19 (a) True (p. 90).
   (b) True (p. 90).
   (c) True (p. 90).
   (d) True (p. 90).
   (e) False (p. 90): delusions and hallucinations commonly occur in the course of dementia but are not indicative of depression.

   Note. Other signs include sad appearance, early wakening, loss of appetite, diurnal variation in mood, loss of interest in surroundings.

20 (a) True (p. 110).
   (b) True (p. 110): in later life the female:male ratio is 7:3.
   (c) False (p. 110): hyperactivity and dysregulation.
   (d) True (p. 110).
   (e) True (p. 110): includes night-time wakefulness and decreases in slow-wave sleep, total REM sleep and REM latency.

21 (a) True (p. 149).
   (b) True (p. 149).
   (c) True (p. 149).
   (d) True (p. 149).
   (e) False (p. 149): tactile hallucinations are less common but not rare.

22 (a) True (p. 150).
   (b) True (p. 150).
   (c) True (p. 150).
   (d) True (p. 150).
   (e) True (p. 150).

   Note. Also persecution, reference and hypochondriasis.

23  The following symptoms are uncommon in late paraphrenia:
(a)  Thought disorder.
(b)  Catatonic symptoms.
(c)  Negative symptoms.
(d)  Delusions of sin.
(e)  Olfactory hallucinations.

24  Risk factors for late paraphrenia include:
(a)  Female gender.
(b)  Degenerative hearing impairment.
(c)  Social isolation.
(d)  Brain disease.
(e)  Family history of schizophreniform disorder.

25  Deep white matter lesions are found in:
(a)  Depression.
(b)  Multi-infarct dementia.
(c)  Multiple sclerosis.
(d)  Hydrocephalus.
(e)  Binswanger's disease.

26  The following occur in the elderly:
(a)  Increased levels of free drugs.
(b)  Increased half-life of psychotropic drugs.
(c)  Increased concentration of water-soluble compounds.
(d)  Glomerular filtration reduces by up to half by the age of 70 years.
(e)  Significant changes in absorption.

27  The following are recognised psychological therapies for dementia:
(a)  Reality orientation.
(b)  Reminiscence.
(c)  Validation therapy.
(d)  Resolution therapy.
(e)  Memory therapy.

23  (a)  True (p. 150).
    (b)  True (p. 150).
    (c)  True (p. 150).
    (d)  True (p. 150).
    (e)  True (p. 150).

24  (a)  True (p. 153): the female:male ratio is in the range 3:1 to 20:1.
    (b)  False (pp. 153–154): conductive rather than degenerative hearing impairment.
    (c)  True (p. 154). Being single is also a risk factor.
    (d)  True (p. 154).
    (e)  True (p. 154).

25  (a)  True (p. 188).
    (b)  True (p. 188).
    (c)  True (p. 188).
    (d)  True (p. 188).
    (e)  True (p. 188).

26  (a)  True (p. 247): because of decreased plasma proteins/albumin.
    (b)  True (p. 247): because of increased body fat (fat acts as a reservoir for psychotropic drugs).
    (c)  True (p. 247): because of a reduction in body water.
    (d)  True (p. 247).
    (e)  False (p. 247): absorption is not grossly affected.

27  (a)  True (p. 272): reality orientation focuses on disorientation and impaired short-term memory.
    (b)  True (p. 273).
    (c)  True (p. 274): validation therapy focuses on the phenomenology of dementia at an emotional rather than a factual level.
    (d)  True (p. 275): resolution therapy is a companion to reality orientation. It looks for meaning in the 'here and now' in the behaviour and confused talk of patients with dementia.
    (e)  True (p. 274).

# Index

## Compiled by Linda English

241

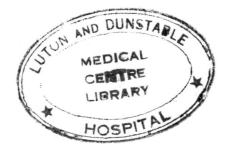